Contents

Preface to the Third Edition

This revised, revamped and updated edition of the popular PasTest title *Surgical Finals: Structured Answer and Essay Questions* employs a unique approach to the presentation of surgical core cases. In this new edition, entitled *Surgical Finals: Short Cases with Structured Answers*, the information is presented in an interactive format which enables the reader to more effectively synthesise and integrate the information. The text covers the complete syllabus of surgery in general and allied subspecialties, including orthopaedics and trauma, neurosurgery, eye, ENT, skin, endocrinology, breast, urology, and vascular surgery. Two new chapters - cardiothoracic surgery and ICU and anaesthesia and several new cases in other chapters have been included in this expanded edition. The text itself consists of 166 clinical scenarios, with each case presented initially as an unknown clinical problem.

In Part I, the reader is presented with a case-based review of common surgical patients. Clinical vignettes or scenarios presenting common surgical conditions are followed by short questions covering the aetiology, pathogenesis and pathology, clinical features, differential diagnosis and management of these surgical conditions.

In Part II, model answers to the questions in Part I provide the reader with a interactive case-based discussion of the disease processes. Additional cogent information is also presented here as 'comment'. This is either relevant to the disease entity or to the management, or both.

Part III offers the reader advice on how to approach essay questions through structured outlines and model essays. Part IV contains a selection of typical essay questions for essay writing practice, and three appendices follow - containing material likely to be helpful to the reader. New for this edition is the Index of Cases - included for quick reference and cross referencing.

Although the book, as the title suggests, is mainly intended for undergraduates preparing for their finals it can also be used by Foundation years in surgery and surgical trainees of basic surgery preparing for the MRCS examinations. It is expected that this unique case-based review of surgery will enable all students of surgery to enhance their knowledge, and will prove a useful method of self-assessment for the reader to check their progress at each stage of the surgical course.

This new edition may be used in one of two ways: as a testing tool to sharpen one's knowledge of an "unknown" clinical problem, or as an information resource of an encapsulated but complete review of a given surgical subject.

Revision Checklist

Use this checklist to record your revision progress. Tick the subjects when you feel confident that you have covered them adequately. This will ensure that you do not forget to revise any key topics.

Chapter 1: Surgical Physiology
☐ Fluid and electrolyte therapy
☐ Acid–base balance
☐ Enteral and parenteral feeding
☐ Transfusion reactions

Chapter 2: Trauma and Burns
☐ ATLS
☐ Head injury assessment
☐ Cervical spine injury
☐ Thoracic injury
☐ Blunt abdominal trauma
☐ Fracture of pelvis and long bones
☐ Assessment of burns
☐ Colloid and crystalloid therapy in burns

Chapter 3: Orthopaedics
☐ Osteoarthritis of the hip
☐ Rheumatoid arthritis
☐ Osteomyelitis
☐ Bone tumours
☐ Kyphoscoliosis

Chapter 4: Neurosurgery
☐ Head injury
☐ Meningomyelocele
☐ Hydrocephalus
☐ Hypothalamic/pituitary lesions
☐ Peripheral nerve injuries

Chapter 5: Skin, Eyes and ENT
☐ Melanoma
☐ Squamous carcinoma
☐ Basal cell carcinoma
☐ The painful red eye
☐ Retinoblastoma
☐ Glaucoma
☐ Uveitis
☐ Tonsillitis
☐ Nose bleed
☐ Chronic sinusitis
☐ Otitis media

Chapter 6: Endocrinology and Breast
☐ Toxic goitre
☐ Thyroid malignancy
☐ Parathyroid hyperplasia

Recommended Reading

General surgical texts

Clinical Examination of the Patient
Lumley JSP and Bouloux PMG, Hodder Arnold, 1994
This book, with 486 colour photographs, serves as a useful guide
for formulating and perfecting examination techniques.

Hamilton Bailey's Physical Signs

Demonstration of Physical Signs in Surgery, 18th Rev edn
Lumley JSP (ed.), Hodder Arnold, 1997
The recent edition of this well-known book on clinical diagnosis
contains many new illustrations on the spectrum of surgical
diseases and highlights the salient features of their diagnosis.

Demonstrations of Physical Signs in Clinical Surgery: Picture tests
18th Rev edn
JSP Lumley, S Chan, H Harris and MOM Zongana, Butterworth-
Heinemann, 2000

Surgery Minitext
Lumley JSP, Scrodon P, Visvanathan R, Hodder Arnold 2004
A concise guide to the management of the surgical patient with a
comprehensive coverage of the generality of surgery contained in a
readily accessible format.

Bailey and Love's New Short Practice of Surgery, 22nd Rev edn
Mann CV, Russell RCG and Williams NS, Hodder Arnold, 1999
A complete reference textbook that forms the basis of surgery after
the finals.

Orthopaedic texts

Essentials of Orthopaedic Examination, 3rd edn
Hammer A, Edward Arnold, 1994

A small, clearly illustrated book that adopts a systematic approach to its examination schemes.

Concise System of Orthopaedics and Fractures, 2nd Rev edn
Apley AG and Solomon L, Butterworth Heinemann, 1994

A standard orthopaedics book, full of useful sketches, photographs and radiographs that bring the text to life. It contains examination schemes for different joints. The recent edition has been extensively updated and includes new illustrations.

Abbreviations

A&E	accident and emergency department
ABG	arterial blood gases estimation
ABPI	ankle brachial pressure index
ACTH	adrenocorticotrophin
ADH	antidiuretic hormone
AIDS	acquired immune deficiency syndrome
AP	anteroposterior
AS	aortic stenosis
ATLS	Advanced Trauma Life Support Systems
AV	atrioventricular
BCC	basal cell cancer
BP	blood pressure
Ca^{2+}	calcium ion
CABG	coronary artery bypass grafting
CAE	carcinoembryonic antigen
Cl^-	chloride ions
CO_2	carbon dioxide
COPD	chronic obstructive pulmonary disease
CPB	cardiopulmonary bypass
CRP	C-reative protein
CSF	cerebrospinal fluid
CSOM	chronic suppurative otitis media
CT	computed tomography
CVP	central venous pressure
DVT	deep vein thrombosis
ECG	electrocardiogram
EDH	extradural haematoma
EEG	electroencephalogram
ERCP	endoscopic retrograde cholangiopancreatography
ESR	erythrocyte sedimentation rate
FBC	full blood count
FEV_1	forced expiratory volume in 1 second
FNAC	fine-needle aspiration cytology

FFP	fresh-frozen plasma
FVC	forced vital capacity
GCS	Glasgow Coma Scale
GI	gastrointestinal
GORD	gastro-oesophageal reflux disease
H^+	proton or hydrogen ion
H_2O	water
Hb	haemoglobin
HCO_3^-	bicarbonate ion
HDU	high dependency unit
HIV	human immunodeficiency virus
ICP	intracranial pressure
ICU	intensive care unit
INR	international normalised ratio
IVU	intravenous urography
JVP	jugular venous pressure
K^+	potassium ion
kcal	kilocalorie
KCl	potassium chloride
kg	kilogramme
kPa	kilopascals
KUB	kidneys, ureter and bladder
l	litre
LAD	left anterior descending
LFT	liver function test
LOS	lower oesophageal sphincter
LV	left ventricle
ml	millilitre
Mg^{2+}	magnesium ion
MIBG	metaiodobenzylguanidine
MRI	magnetic resonance imaging
Na^+	sodium ion
NaCl	sodium chloride
NEC	necrotising enterocolitis
NPO	nil per oris
NSAIDs	non-steroidal anti-inflammatory drugs

NSCLC	non-small-cell lung cancer
O_2	oxygen
OGD	oesophagogastroduodenoscopy
PCV	packed cell volume
PO_4^{3-}	phosphate ion
PPF	plasma protein fraction
PT	prothrombin time
PTA	percutaneous transluminal angioplasty
PTC	percutaneous transhepatic cholangiogram
PTH	parathyroid hormone
SDH	subdural haematoma
SMRP	serum mesothelin-related protein
T_3	tri-iodothyronine
T_4	thyroxine
TB	tuberculosis
tPA	tissue plasminogen activator
TSH	thyroid-stimulating hormone
U&Es	urea and electrolytes
WBC	white blood cell count

Dedication

In memory of our fathers
JSPL, RV
To my parents
SGR

PART ONE

Structured Answer Questions

1

Surgical Physiology

Question 1

A 49-year-old man with a history of macronodular cirrhosis is admitted for elective gastrointestinal surgery. His liver biochemistry is as follows:
- *Conjugated bilirubin: 25 μmol/l*
- *Alkaline phosphatase: 760 units/l*
- *Serum albumin: 15 g/l*
- *Aspartate and alanine aminotransferases: elevated*
- *Plasma prothrombin index: decreased*
- *Gamma glutamyltransferase (GGT): raised*

(a) Comment on his liver profile *(4 marks)*

(b) How would you support his liver function before surgery? *(3 marks)*

(c) List three surgical complications associated with the above dysfunction *(3 marks)*

Question 2

A 67-year-old man with chronic lung disease is admitted for preoperative assessment for elective abdominal surgery. His lung function tests are as follows:
- *Peak expiratory flow rate (PEFR): 350 l/min (normal: 400–600 l/min)*
- *Forced expiratory volume in 1 second (FEV_1): 2.2 l (normal: 3.2 l)*
- *Forced vital capacity (FVC): 4.2 l (normal: 4.0–5.5 l)*
- *Po_2: 7.8 kPa (normal: 10.6 kPa)*
- *Pco_2: 6.98 kPa (normal: 4.6–6.4 kPa)*

(a) Comment on his respiratory impairment   *(4 marks)*

(b) Outline measures to improve lung function before surgery   *(3 marks)*

(c) How would you support his respiratory function in the postoperative period?   *(3 marks)*

Question 3

A 70-year-old man is assessed for an emergency laparotomy for peritonitis caused by colonic diverticular perforation. He passes 45 ml urine over the subsequent 2 h; his peripheral blood count and serum biochemistry are as follows:
- Hb: 9.8 g/l
- White blood cell count (WBC): 21.4 × 10^6 cells/mm^3
- Na$^+$: 145 mmol/l
- K$^+$: 5.6 mmol/l
- HCO$_3^-$: 30 mmol/l
- Urea: 60 mmol/l

(a) (i) Comment on his biochemical profile *(2 marks)*

(ii) List the causes of renal malfunction in this patient
(2 marks)

(b) Outline how renal function may be improved before surgery *(2 marks)*

(c) State a renal complication of surgery and anaesthesia, and outline your management *(4 marks)*

Question 4

A 78-year-old man weighing 53 kg is admitted from a nursing home with a 14-day history of persistent vomiting. He is very dehydrated and malnourished.

(a) (i) How would you estimate his fluid and electrolyte deficit? *(1 mark)*

(ii) List the fluid and electrolyte preparations that you would use, with their approximate compositions, to correct his deficit *(2 marks)*

(iii) How would you monitor his fluid replacement therapy? *(2 marks)*

(b) (i) How would you assess his state of nutrition? *(2 marks)*

(ii) Discuss briefly how you would work out his protein and calorie requirements *(3 marks)*

Question 5

A 65-year-old man is admitted with a 3-day history of vomiting and a diagnosis of gastric outlet obstruction is made. He is placed on nasogastric aspiration and an intravenous infusion of 5% dextrose, alternating with Hartmann's (Ringer's lactate) solution over the next 48 h. His serum biochemistry on admission was: Na^+ 120 mmol/l, K^+ 3.7 mmol/l, HCO_3^- 40 mmol/l. His urinary pH at the end of this period is 7.2.

(a) (i) State the biochemical diagnosis on admission *(1 mark)*

(ii) Comment on the fluid and electrolyte replacement that followed *(3 marks)*

(b) Write a note on the metabolic factors responsible for the production of acidic urine *(6 marks)*

Question 6

A 60-year-old man underwent elective abdominal surgery for repair of an aortic aneurysm.

(a) (i) What is the metabolic response with respect to fluid and electrolyte balance in the first 24 hours of surgery? *(2 marks)*

(ii) How would you adjust the fluid and electrolyte requirements during this period? *(2 marks)*

(b) His urine output fell to below 30 ml/h after surgery:

(i) How would you determine the cause of his oliguria? *(4 marks)*

(ii) What remedial measures would you take? *(2 marks)*

Question 7

A man became pyrexial and developed an erythematous skin rash during a blood transfusion after surgery.

(a) (i) What factors are involved in these reactions? *(2 marks)*

(ii) What measures would you take to counteract these complications? *(2 marks)*

(b) In the postoperative period the patient required a 10-unit blood transfusion:

(i) What is the effect of this transfusion on liver function and clotting factors? *(2 marks)*

(ii) What is the effect on plasma potassium and calcium levels and how would you achieve homoeostasis of these ions in the plasma? *(4 marks)*

Question 8

A 34-year-old man with advanced infection with the human immunodeficiency virus (HIV) develops a bowel obstruction that requires emergency surgery.

(a) (i) List the changes in the haematological or biochemical parameters that would, in the perioperative period, make him susceptible to haemorrhage *(2 marks)*

(ii) List the haematological or biochemical changes, in the perioperative period, that would make him susceptible to infection *(3 marks)*

(b) (i) State the measures taken to protect theatre personnel from accidental inoculation with a patient's body fluids with regard to wearing protective garb *(2 marks)*

(ii) What important measures should be taken with regard to safety in surgical instrument usage? *(3 marks)*

Question 9

A 43-year-old woman suffering from diabetes mellitus is admitted as an emergency with gangrene of the toes of her left foot. She was drowsy and her arterial blood gas (ABG) estimation revealed a pH of 7.1 and a P_{CO_2} of 6.8 kPa.

(a) (i) State which acid–base disorder is present *(1 mark)*

(ii) Give two causes for this *(2 marks)*

(b) (i) State further investigations that you would request *(3 marks)*

(ii) How would you manage the metabolic disorder? *(4 marks)*

Question 10

A 49-year-old man with a malignant stricture of the oesophagus had lost 20% of his normal body weight over a 5-month period.

(a) (i) State the cause of his weight loss *(1 mark)*

(ii) How would you categorise his nutritional state? *(1 mark)*

(iii) List two clinical findings that would reflect the nutritional state *(2 marks)*

(b) (i) How would you improve his nutritional state? *(3 marks)*

(ii) How would you monitor your nutrition therapy? *(3 marks)*

Question 11

A 28-year-old man involved in a bar fight suffered an 8-cm-long, muscle-deep incisional wound on his forearm.

(a) List three local factors affecting the healing of this wound *(3 marks)*

(b) List three systemic factors affecting the healing of this wound *(3 marks)*

(c) List the complications of wound healing *(4 marks)*

Trauma and Burns

Question 1

A 30-year-old man is brought to the Emergency Department having sustained a closed head injury from a blow to the back of the head.

(a) How would you assess the level of consciousness?

(2 marks)

(b) List the physical signs that you would elicit to establish the extent of the intracranial injury *(3 marks)*

(c) (i) List the types of intracranial bleeding that may be present and state one investigation that would demonstrate the lesion *(2 marks)*

(ii) Write a short note on your management *(3 marks)*

Question 2

A 23-year-old motorcyclist sustained chest injuries in a road accident and was air-lifted to the Emergency Department.

(a) State your immediate measures to assess and maintain respiratory and circulatory function *(3 marks)*

(b) Identify two immediately life-threatening intrathoracic emergencies during your primary clinical survey *(2 marks)*

(c) Write a note on the management of:
   (i)   An open chest wound *(2 marks)*
   (ii) A haemopneumothorax *(3 marks)*

Question 3

A driver of a motor vehicle involved in a head-on collision with another vehicle was air-lifted to the Emergency Department fully conscious and communicative but becoming increasingly breathless, with central cyanosis and bruising over his right upper chest.

(a) (i) State the two probable causes for his progressive respiratory failure *(2 marks)*
    (ii) List the clinical signs you would elicit to confirm your diagnoses *(2 marks)*

(b) (i) State one blood investigation that you would urgently request *(1 mark)*
    (ii) State the radiological investigations that would confirm the diagnosis *(1 mark)*

(c) State four potentially lethal thoracic injuries that he may have sustained, which may not be apparent during the initial clinical survey *(4 marks)*

Question 4

A 43-year-old woman fell off her horse in a riding accident. She complains of severe and persistent upper abdominal pain radiating to her back.

(a) (i) List the possible intra-abdominal visceral injuries sustained *(2 marks)*

  (ii) State one non-invasive investigation that you would perform to assess the presence and extent of an intra-abdominal injury *(1 mark)*

(b) (i) How would you monitor this patient in the Emergency Department?

(2 marks)

  (ii) What are the immediate resuscitatory measures that you may be called upon to perform? *(2 marks)*

(c) Discuss the clinical and other findings that would require an emergency surgical exploration of the abdomen *(3 marks)*

Question 5

You are a member of an air ambulance team attending a 28-year-old man with multiple injuries at the site of a road traffic accident.

(a) State in order of priority your measures to ensure patient survival until transfer to a trauma centre

(5 marks)

(b) The patient is trapped in the wreckage of his vehicle and his transfer is delayed by 3 hours. Discuss your supportive measures *(3 marks)*

(c) List the ideal composition of an air ambulance team

(2 marks)

Question 6

An 18-year-old motorcyclist involved in a road traffic accident was admitted to the Emergency Department. He is fully conscious but complains of severe neck pain.

(a) List the possible injuries to the cervical spine and cervical cord that he may have sustained *(2 marks)*

(b) When gently examining the neck:

(i) What findings would suggest a spinal injury? *(1 mark)*

(ii) What manoeuvre should you not perform? *(1 mark)*

(c) If he were found to have a spinal fracture and cord lesion at the C5–T1 level:

(i) Discuss your treatment of the injury *(2 marks)*

(ii) How would you prevent complications as sequelae to the injury? *(4 marks)*

Question 7

An 8-year-old girl suffered hot water scalds to the whole of her chest and abdomen. She is admitted to the Emergency Department conscious and very distressed.

(a) (i) How would you estimate the surface area affected? *(1 mark)*

(ii) State the immediate medical measures that you would take *(4 marks)*

(b) (i) How would you distinguish between a partial-thickness and a full-thickness skin burn? *(2 marks)*

(ii) How would you calculate the fluid replacement for the first 24 hours? *(3 marks)*

Question 8

A 30-year-old secretary was rescued from an office fire. She is breathless and coughing, with traces of soot around her nose and mouth. She had suffered no external burns.

(a) (i)   State the injury sustained   *(1 mark)*

(ii) Give your immediate resuscitation measures
                                                                    (2 marks)

(b) She develops stridor and respiratory distress:

(i)   State the pathological process involved   *(2 marks)*

(ii) How would you manage her airway?   *(2 marks)*

(iii) How would you treat the injury sustained?
                                                                    (3 marks)

Question 9

A 20-year-old man injured his neck when the scrum collapsed on him while playing rugby.

(a) (i)   How would you avoid compounding a suspected spinal injury?   *(2 marks)*

(ii) How would you investigate for the integrity of the cervical spine?   *(2 marks)*

(b) If the patient is unconscious, list the clinical findings that suggest a cervical cord injury   *(3 marks)*

(c) Write a note on neurogenic shock following cervical cord injury   *(3 marks)*

Question 10

A 15-year-old cyclist was admitted to the Emergency Department following a traffic accident. He is conscious but very pale, with bruising over the right lower chest and abdomen, and a swelling of the right thigh and knee.

(a) How would you assess for the following:

    (i) Lung injury   *(2 marks)*

    (ii) Intra-abdominal injury   *(2 marks)*

    (iii) Lower limb injury   *(2 marks)*

(b) He develops hypovolaemic shock. List your immediate measures to resuscitate him   *(4 marks)*

Question 11

A 5-year-old boy was seen in the Emergency Department, having sustained hot water scalds to his arms, chest and abdomen at home.

(a) How would you determine the extent and depth of his wounds on examination?   *(3 marks)*

(b) State your criteria for admission   *(3 marks)*

(c) Write a note on the methods of dressing his wounds   *(4 marks)*

Question 12

A 38-year-old railway worker is admitted to the Emergency Department with electrical burns to his back and arm, from contact with high-tension overhead conductors.

(a) State three urgent priorities in his clinical assessment
(3 marks)

(b) Write a note on the type of burn injury sustained
(3 marks)

(c) Discuss the effect of the injury on the heart, kidneys, skeletal muscle and nervous system *(4 marks)*

Question 13

A 49-year-old motorist sustained burns to 35% of his body surface from burning fuel in a traffic accident.

(a) How would you estimate his fluid requirements for the first 24 hours? *(3 marks)*

(b) What measures would you take to prevent wound infection? *(4 marks)*

(c) How would you manage a non-survivable burn injury?
(3 marks)

Question 14

Five patients injured in a single motor vehicle accident are admitted to the Emergency Department. They are:

- *Patient 1: an 18-year-old front-seat passenger found 10 m from the vehicle. He is awake and complains of severe chest and limb pains; there are angulated deformities of the left forearm and left thigh; his BP is 90/60 mmHg, pulse 140 beats/min and respiration 35/min.*
- *Patient 2: a 19-year-old man, found in the driving seat of the vehicle, is unconscious with severe facial bruising and bleeding from the nose and mouth; there are multiple abrasions over the anterior chest wall; his BP is 150/80 mmHg, pulse 120 beats/min and respiration 40/min.*
- *Patient 3: a 20-year-old hysterical woman extracted from the floor of the back seat complains of abdominal pains; she is 8 months pregnant and is found to be in active labour; her vital signs are normal.*
- *Patient 4: a 16-year-old girl, a back-seat passenger, complains of severe neck pain and paraesthesiae of both arms and hands; her vital signs are normal.*
- *Patient 5: a 17-year-old girl, a back-seat passenger, complains of pain in her right hip and both feet; she has bruising and deformities of both ankles; her vital signs are normal.*

(a) In what order would you care for these patients? Place them in descending order of priority *(3 marks)*

(b) Briefly outline your reasons for prioritising the patients thus *(7 marks)*

Question 15

A hurricane with heavy rains caused a mudslide, burying a section of a hillside village. Five villagers were rescued 10 hours later. They are:

- *Patient 1: a 44-year-old man found buried in mud; he is comatose with weak peripheral pulses, and there are open wounds over the shoulder and back that are not actively bleeding.*
- *Patient 2: a 34-year-old woman who fell 10 m down a precipice; she is awake but very lethargic with a large laceration in her scalp that is actively bleeding.*
- *Patient 3: a 13-year-old girl found pinned under a fallen tree; she is awake and alert and complains of pain in both legs and numbness of her feet; she has swelling, bruising and angulated deformities of the right knee and left leg.*
- *Patient 4: a 29-year-old woman, who dug herself out from under the mud, is increasingly breathless and complains of right-sided chest and abdominal pain; paradoxical movement is observed over the right chest.*
- *Patient 5: a 9-year-old girl, found wandering near the mud slide, is distressed and confused but appears not to be in pain and to have no external injuries.*

(a) In what order would you care for these patients? Place them in descending order of priority *(3 marks)*

(b) Briefly outline your reasons for prioritising the patients thus *(7 marks)*

Question 16

Five holidaymakers were admitted to the Emergency Department 2 hours after a gas cylinder explosion and fire in a caravan at a seaside resort. They are:

- *Patient 1: a 38-year-old man with 60% full- and partial-thickness surface burns to the anterior aspect of his torso and limbs; he has a large laceration in the scalp and is expectorating carbonaceous sputum; his BP is 130/100 mmHg, pulse 120/min and respiration 30/min.*
- *Patient 2: a 32-year-old woman, with 25% full- and partial-thickness burns to the chest and arms and forearms, complains of severe neck pains and has bruising and a deformity of her left shoulder; her BP is 120/90 mmHg, pulse 100/min and respiration 28/min.*
- *Patient 3: a 72-year-old woman, with 65% surface burns to the face, chest, upper abdomen and arms, is semi-comatose with sonorous breathing; her BP is 110/90 mmHg, pulse 125/min and respiration 14/min.*
- *Patient 4: a 12-year-old boy, with 15% mostly superficial burns, is found to have deep lacerations to his left hip and thigh that are actively bleeding; his BP is 90/60 mmHg, pulse 130/min and respiration 28/min.*
- *Patient 5: a 5-year-old girl was found confused and lethargic with soot over her nose and mouth, and had sustained no external injuries; her BP is 110/70 mmHg, pulse 110/min and respiration 32/min.*

(a) In what order would you care for these patients? Place them in descending order of priority   *(3 marks)*

(b) Briefly outline your reasons for prioritising the patients thus   *(7 marks)*

Question 17

You are the casualty officer in an Emergency Department when you are informed by the police that a passenger aircraft has overshot the runway on landing and caught fire at the local airport 15 miles from your local hospital. Casualties are being taken to three hospitals in the area and you are to expect the arrival of some of them.

(a) List the hospital personnel whom you need to contact immediately   *(3 marks)*

(b) List the parts of the hospital that you would designate as reception and treatment areas   *(3 marks)*

(c) What categories of triage would you use for the incoming casualties?   *(4 marks)*

Question 18

A 43-year-old man was struck by a motorcycle, while crossing the road. He fell on the road and was unable to stand up without support. He complained of severe pain in his pubic region. Examination on arrival in the Emergency Department revealed blood at the tip of the penis and tenderness over the pelvis with pelvic springing. No other clinical findings were elicited on examination of the head, neck, thorax, abdomen and limbs.

(a) What is the most likely diagnosis?   *(2 marks)*

(b) What other clinical signs may be elicited in such an injury?   *(4 marks)*

(c) What immediate complications are associated with such an injury?   *(2 marks)*

(d) What will be the investigation of choice in such a case?
                                                   (2 marks)

3 Orthopaedics

Question 1

A 14-year-old child presents with pain over a swelling of 3 months' duration, arising from the lower end of the femur.

(a) State two investigations that would assist in the diagnosis *(2 marks)*

(b) List three bone tumours that may present at this age *(3 marks)*

(c) Outline the principles of treating bone tumours in childhood *(5 marks)*

Question 2

A 33-year-old, otherwise healthy, woman presents with a 9-month history of progressive pain in her lower back, which is worse after activity; over the past few weeks she developed tingling sensations and numbness in the left leg.

(a) Outline the probable cause of her symptoms and state the likely diagnosis *(3 marks)*

(b) How would you identify the site or level of the lesion by neurological assessment? *(3 marks)*

(c) Outline the principles of treating this condition *(4 marks)*

Question 3

A 69-year-old woman develops increasing pain and stiffness in the hip 6 months after hip joint replacement on that side.

(a) List three causes for her symptoms   *(3 marks)*

(b) How would you assess her symptoms?   *(3 marks)*

(c) Outline the factors that contribute to the complications of joint replacement surgery   *(4 marks)*

Question 4

A 61-year-old woman complains of swelling, pain and inflammation of her bunions, which for many years have been the cause of unsightly deformity of her feet.

(a) (i) State your diagnosis   *(2 marks)*

(ii) List the factors responsible for her symptoms   *(2 marks)*

(b) State the predisposing cause of this deformity   *(2 marks)*

(c) Outline the surgical treatment of this condition   *(4 marks)*

Question 5

A 44-year-old woman gives a 6-month history of progressive pain in her neck on movement, after a mild whiplash injury. In recent weeks she has experienced numbness and weakness in her right hand.

(a) State the probable diagnosis and the causative factors
(3 marks)

(b) How would you assess the segmental level of the neurological lesion? *(3 marks)*

(c) Outline the principles of treating this condition
(4 marks)

Question 6

A 9-year-old schoolgirl presents at the orthopaedic clinic with a 4-month history of pain in her left groin and hip, and a progressive limp. She gives no history of trauma or other symptoms.

(a) List the positive findings that you would expect on examining her hip *(3 marks)*

(b) (i) State two diseases that may present thus at this age
(2 marks)

(ii) List the radiological features that you would expect to see in each *(2 marks)*

(c) What are their complications if left untreated? *(3 marks)*

Question 7

A 17-year-old schoolboy sustained an external rotational injury to his right ankle during a rugby tackle. There was considerable pain, bruising and swelling.

(a) List the possible injuries to the ankle *(4 marks)*

(b) Radiology of the ankle and distal tibia and fibula showed no fracture. What related bony and/or ligamentous injuries would you wish to exclude?

(2 marks)

(c) Write a note on the treatment of an unstable ankle injury *(4 marks)*

Question 8

A 40-year-old woman suffered with pain, swelling and loss of mobility in her fingers, which over a period of time affected her wrists and feet.

(a) (i) State the likely diagnosis *(1 mark)*

(ii) Write a note on the pathological changes in the joints *(3 marks)*

(b) List the positive blood investigations in this disease *(3 marks)*

(c) State the principles of management *(3 marks)*

Question 9

A 64-year-old woman with pain, stiffness and limitation of movement in her left hip is diagnosed as having osteoarthritis.

(a) List the radiological features in the hip joint   *(3 marks)*

(b) State non-surgical measures to alleviate symptoms and preserve function   *(3 marks)*

(c) (i) List the indications for surgical treatment
         (3 marks)

    (ii) State the operation of choice for this patient
         (1 mark)

Question 10

A 6-year-old boy sustained a supracondylar fracture to his right arm during a fall in the school playground.

(a) Write a note on the treatment of the fracture   *(4 marks)*

(b) Eight hours after the fracture was reduced, the child is crying with severe pain and unable to grasp objects with the right hand. The forearm is swollen and the radial pulse absent. Write a note on your diagnosis and treatment   *(3 marks)*

(c) List the complications of this fracture   *(3 marks)*

Question 11

A 76-year-old woman is brought to the Emergency Department following a fall on the outstretched right hand. On arrival she has a 'dinner fork' deformity of the right wrist and swelling. She also complains of numbness of the right hand.

(a) What is the most likely injury sustained by this woman?
(1 mark)

(b) What associated injuries must be looked for when someone sustains such an injury? *(3 marks)*

(c) What will be seen on the radiograph in this case?
(3 marks)

(d) What complications may be seen after this injury?
(3 marks)

Question 12

A 19-year-old woman was seen in the surgical outpatient clinic complaining of pain in the big toe of her left foot. She said that the pain worsens with weight bearing and ambulation. On examination she had a swollen, red, tender big toe with friable granulation tissue along the lateral nail margin.

(a) What is the most likely diagnosis? *(1 mark)*

(b) List three causes for this condition *(3 marks)*

(c) What is the pathophysiology of this condition?
(2 marks)

(c) What is the role of radiology in the management of this condition? *(2 marks)*

(d) How will you manage this condition? *(2 marks)*

Question 13

A 53-year-old man with complaints of chronic low back and perineal pain, and a year-long history of difficulty initiating micturition, presented in the Emergency Department with acute urinary retention. On clinical examination he had tenderness in his sacral spine with saddle anaesthesia and loss of bulbocavernosus and anal reflexes.

(a) What is the most likely diagnosis? *(1 mark)*

(b) List three causes for this condition *(3 marks)*

(c) What is the pathophysiology of this condition? *(3 marks)*

(d) Discuss the management of this condition? *(3 marks)*

Question 14

A newborn female baby with breech presentation was assessed by the neonatologist after birth. On examination of her lower limbs the neonatologist elicited a loud 'clunk' from the right hip as the head of the femur reduced into the acetabulum, with the hip in the abducted position.

(a) Write a note on how you would diagnose and treat this condition of the hip in the neonatal period *(5 marks)*

(b) List the factors that give rise to this condition *(2 marks)*

(c) If the diagnosis is delayed until the child starts walking, discuss the treatment options and prognosis *(3 marks)*

Question 15

A child aged 5 years presents to her family practitioner with a 3-day history of severe pain in her left forearm, with fever and malaise. The forearm is inflamed and swollen.

(a) (i) State the probable diagnosis   *(1 mark)*

    (ii) Write a note on the investigations that would aid the diagnosis   *(3 marks)*

(b) Give three differential diagnoses of the forearm swelling   *(3 marks)*

(c) Outline your treatment   *(3 marks)*

Question 16

A boy of 8 years is referred from a child welfare clinic with a growth curve well below the normal range. Clinically there is thickening of his wrists and ankles, and bowing of his legs.

(a) (i) State the likely clinical diagnosis   *(1 mark)*

    (ii) List the radiological features that would confirm your diagnosis   *(2 marks)*

    (iii) List the biochemical features that would confirm your diagnosis   *(2 marks)*

(b) (i) State the causative factors   *(3 marks)*

    (ii) Outline the treatment   *(2 marks)*

Question 17

A 60-year-old man presents with long-standing dull pain in his back and hips, and is found to be of short stature, with kyphosis of the spine and slight forward bowing of his legs.

(a) (i) State the probable clinical diagnosis *(1 mark)*

  (ii) Discuss the bony changes that characterise this disease *(4 marks)*

(b) List four complications of this disease *(2 marks)*

(c) Write a note on the principles of treatment *(3 marks)*

Question 18

A 47-year-old factory worker presents with a painless, fluctuant swelling in his right groin. A kyphotic angulation of the dorsal spine is observed on examination.

(a) (i) State the probable diagnosis *(1 mark)*

  (ii) Discuss the pathological basis of the clinical findings *(2 marks)*

(b) List the investigations to confirm your diagnosis *(3 marks)*

(c) (i) Discuss your objectives in treatment *(3 marks)*

  (ii) State a serious complication that may be precipitated in this patient *(1 mark)*

Question 19

A 5-year-old child suffering from protein–calorie malnutrition presents with an inflamed, swollen and painful forearm of 4 days' duration.

(a) (i) State two lesions that may present thus *(2 marks)*

(ii) How would movements in that limb be affected? *(2 marks)*

(b) (i) List the common organisms that are implicated *(2 marks)*

(ii) Discuss the treatment of these two lesions *(4 marks)*

4

Neurosurgery

Question 1

A 15-year-old boy falls while skateboarding and strikes the left side of his head against a concrete retaining wall. Only a minor scalp abrasion is present at the site of the impact, with minimal bleeding that stops in a few minutes. He is initially alert following this accident, but then became unconscious about 30 minutes later. In the hospital, a head computed tomography (CT) scan reveals a convex, lens-shaped area of haemorrhage centred over the left parietal region.

(a) What is the most likely diagnosis?   *(1 mark)*

(b) Which vessel is commonly involved in such an injury?   *(1 mark)*

(c) Discuss the pathophysiology of this injury   *(4 marks)*

(d) Outline the management of this injury   *(2 marks)*

(e) What is the prognosis of this injury?   *(2 marks)*

Question 2

*A 46-year-old man involved in a head-on collision between two cars was brought to the Emergency Department unconscious. On clinical examination his Glasgow Coma Scale (GCS) score was **4**. He also had a fractured clavicle and laceration on his right arm. Emergency CT performed, immediately after stabilising him using standard Advanced Trauma Life Support (ATLS) guidelines, revealed a large, crescent-shaped, hyperdense area between the inner table of the skull and the surface of the right cerebral hemisphere.*

(a) What is the most likely diagnosis? *(1 mark)*

(b) What is the pathophysiology of this condition?
(2 marks)

(c) What neurological findings may be elicited in a patient with such an injury? *(4 marks)*

(d) What is the management of this condition
(3 marks)

Question 3

A 31-year-old man, a known HIV carrier, gives a 6-month history of recurrent episodes of paranasal sinusitus and, more recently, of febrile episodes and severe headaches. Clinically, he is found to have right oculomotor nerve palsy, loss of positional sense and an unstable gait.

(a) State the probable diagnosis and the cause of his most recent symptoms *(3 marks)*

(b) State one investigation that would confirm your diagnosis and localise the lesion *(2 marks)*

(c) Outline the treatment of this condition *(5 marks)*

Question 4

A 40-year-old merchant seaman with a 5-month history of headaches, paraesthesiae and progressive weakness in his left lower limb is found to have a glial tumour of the right cerebral hemisphere.

(a) List four glial tumours *(2 marks)*

(b) State a method of confirming the diagnosis *(2 marks)*

(c) Outline the principles of treating cerebral tumours *(6 marks)*

Question 5

A 37-year-old bookmaker gives a 7-year history of fits, associated with blackouts, followed by transient loss of speech and cognitive function, which are poorly controlled on antiepileptic medical treatment.

(a) List three investigations that may localise the seizure focus *(3 marks)*

(b) State the indications for surgical treatment *(4 marks)*

(c) How would you counsel the patient for seizure surgery? *(3 marks)*

Question 6

An 11-month-old boy is referred to the neurosurgical clinic with a history of failure to thrive and achieve milestones. A progressive increase in skull circumference has been noted since birth.

(a)   (i)   State the likely diagnosis   *(1 mark)*

      (ii)   What are the positive clinical findings?   *(2 marks)*

      (iii) State one important investigation to confirm your diagnosis   *(1 mark)*

(b)   (i)   State a common cause for this condition   *(1 mark)*

      (ii)   Give two associated malformations of the central nervous system   *(2 marks)*

(c)   Write a note on the definitive treatment for this condition   *(3 marks)*

Question 7

A 48-year-old woman with a 9-month history of epileptic fits and headaches is found to have focal neurological signs and papilloedema.

(a)   (i)   State your working diagnosis   *(1 mark)*

      (ii)   Discuss briefly the pathophysiology of the abnormal findings   *(3 marks)*

(b)   (i)   State two investigations that would reveal the lesion   *(2 marks)*

      (ii)   Why would a lumbar puncture be contraindicated?   *(1 mark)*

(c)   List three benign and three malignant lesions that would present thus   *(3 marks)*

Question 8

A previously healthy 32-year-old woman was admitted complaining of sudden onset of severe headache, with nausea and vomiting. She was found to be drowsy with neck stiffness.

(a) (i) State the likely diagnosis and the underlying lesion *(2 marks)*

(ii) If her condition deteriorates, state the progressive changes in the clinical findings *(3 marks)*

(b) (i) State one non-invasive investigation to confirm your diagnosis *(1 mark)*

(ii) State your findings on lumbar puncture *(1 mark)*

(c) Write a note on her management *(3 marks)*

Question 9

A conscious 75-year-old woman is admitted with a left hemisphere stroke.

(a) (i) List three prime neurological findings *(2 marks)*

(ii) List four risk factors of stroke *(2 marks)*

(b) The patient's condition deteriorates; outline your immediate management *(6 marks)*

Question 10

A 6-year-old child presents with fever and fits. A cranial CT scan reveals a brain abscess.

(a) How would you arrive at this diagnosis clinically?

(3 marks)

(b) (i)   List four causative organisms *(2 marks)*

    (ii) List two underlying sources of infection that predispose to brain abscess in this child *(2 marks)*

(c) Write a note on specific treatment *(3 marks)*

Question 11

A 56-year-old woman complains of gradual onset of pain in her neck, radiating down her left arm. She also experienced tingling down the limb during neck extension.

(a) List three lesions of the spinal cord and three lesions of the cervical spine that may give rise to her symptoms

(3 marks)

(b) Write a note on the likely neurological findings

(3 marks)

(c) (i)   List the radiological investigations to confirm your diagnosis *(2 marks)*

    (ii) State the principles of treatment *(2 marks)*

5 Skin, Eyes and ENT

Question 1

An 8-year-old Eastern European child is air-lifted from a refugee camp for the treatment of an ulcerating lesion in her left cheek that has exposed the buccal cavity and alveolar margin.

(a) State your diagnosis (*2 marks*)

(b) List the aetiological factors implicated in its causation (*3 marks*)

(c) Outline your treatment priorities in the management of this condition (*5 marks*)

Question 2

A 7-year-old child in equatorial Africa is seen by you, during your overseas elective spell, with a 4-month history of a minimally symptomatic swelling over the cheek bone, deforming her face.

(a) (i) State your probable diagnosis (*2 marks*)
  (ii) Give two investigations to confirm your diagnosis (*2 marks*)

(b) List the aetiological factors associated with this condition (*3 marks*)

(c) How would you treat this lesion? (*3 marks*)

Question 3

A 38-year-old man presents with an unhealed ulcer over a burn scar over the left shin that he sustained 2 years previously

(a) State the likely diagnosis and your clinical findings

(4 marks)

(b) How would you confirm your diagnosis?　　*(2 marks)*

(c) How would you treat this lesion?　　*(4 marks)*

Question 4

A 72-year-old, otherwise fit and healthy, farmer was seen in the surgical outpatient clinic complaining of a non-healing sore of 6 months' duration on his right cheek. He mentioned that minor trauma, such as shaving or drying with a towel, causes bleeding.

(a) What is the most likely diagnosis?　　*(1 mark)*

(b) Name three conditions that may be considered in the differential diagnosis of this lesion?　　*(3 marks)*

(c) How can you confirm the diagnosis?　　*(3 marks)*

(d) Briefly discuss the management of this condition

(3 marks)

Question 5

A 54-year old woman presents with a 12-week history of a circumscribed, 2.5 cm diameter, itchy, ulcerating, pigmented skin lesion on her upper back; it had recently bled.

(a) (i) What are the other clinical features of the lesion that you would look for on examination? *(1 mark)*

(ii) State a malignant lesion that may present thus *(1 mark)*

(iii) How is it staged histologically? *(2 marks)*

(b) How would you treat this lesion? *(3 marks)*

(c) Write a short note on the public health measures that you would adopt to reduce the incidence of this form of skin cancer in the community *(3 marks)*

Question 6

A small, circumscribed, raised lesion on the cheek of an 87-year-old woman bled after minor trauma.

(a) State three malignant lesions that may present thus *(3 marks)*

(b) If your clinical diagnosis is a form of skin cancer, what treatment options are available? *(4 marks)*

(c) (i) Discuss the association of solar radiation with the development of skin lesions *(2 marks)*

(ii) What protective measures would you advise? *(1 mark)*

Question 7

A 70-year-old woman suffers a sudden painless loss of vision in one eye.

(a) Give four possible causes   *(4 marks)*

(b) State three associated systemic diseases   *(3 marks)*

(c) If she had suffered loss of vision in both eyes, state two probable causes   *(3 marks)*

Question 8

A 3-year-old toddler is seen in the Emergency Department with a 5-day history of a painful red eye.

(a) List four possible causes   *(2 marks)*

(b) Write a note on your examination of the eye   *(4 marks)*

(c) If a white pupillary reflex was seen on fundoscopy, state your probable diagnosis and management   *(4 marks)*

Question 9

An 11-year-old boy was admitted with right-sided proptosis, oedematous conjunctivitis (chemosis) and reduced visual acuity. He was found to be pyrexial, dehydrated and lethargic. There was a recent history of recurrent acute sinus infection.

(a) (i) State your clinical diagnosis *(1 mark)*

(ii) What microbiological and radiological investigations would you request? *(2 marks)*

(b) (i) State your medical management of this condition *(2 marks)*

(ii) How would you monitor the response to your medical measures? *(2 marks)*

(c) The child fails to improve, with deterioration in his eye signs. A CT scan shows an opacity of the right maxillary sinus and an abscess under the orbital plate of the ethmoid bone:

(i) State the surgical measures required *(2 marks)*

(ii) State a potentially lethal complication of this condition *(1 mark)*

Question 10

A cricketer fielding close to the wicket was struck in the orbit by a firmly hit cricket ball. He presented to the Emergency Department with periocular ecchymosis and periorbital swelling.

(a) (i) State the probable orbital injury sustained *(1 mark)*

(ii) State the mechanism of the injury to the orbit
(2 marks)

(b) (i) Discuss the positive findings when examining for orbital damage *(3 marks)*

(ii) List the investigations that you would require to exclude bony injury *(1 mark)*

(c) Discuss the principles of managing this injury *(3 marks)*

Question 11

An 11-year-old boy with a 4-year history of recurrent throat infections presents to the Emergency Department with fever, malaise, sore throat and dysphagia.

(a) (i) State the probable diagnosis *(2 marks)*

(ii) What is a frequently accompanying lesion in the nasopharynx? *(2 marks)*

(b) List the findings on examination *(3 marks)*

(c) Outline the definitive treatment for these lesions
(3 marks)

Question 12

A 48-year-old man presents to the ENT clinic with a 6-week history of progressive hoarseness not responding to antibiotics.

(a) List four non-malignant lesions of the vocal folds that may present thus *(2 marks)*

(b) Write a note on two methods of clinically examining the larynx *(4 marks)*

(c) A biopsy of a small lesion on the vocal fold revealed a squamous cell carcinoma (glottic carcinoma). Discuss the treatment options available *(4 marks)*

Question 13

A 50-year-old man is brought to an Emergency Department with an uncontrollable acute nosebleed.

(a) What is the medical term for a nosebleed? *(1 mark)*

(b) How will you classify a nosebleed? *(2 marks)*

(c) List three causes for a nosebleed. *(3 marks)*

(d) Discuss the management of this patient? *(4 marks)*

Question 14

A 23-year-old woman with ear discharge of more than 6 weeks' duration presents in an Emergency Department complaining of loss of hearing. On clinical examination serosanguineous and foul-smelling ear discharge is observed with a perforation in the tympanic membrane. The superior quadrant of the tympanic membrane was obscured by a polyp.

(a) What is the most likely diagnosis? *(2 marks)*

(b) Discuss the aetiology of this condition *(2 marks)*

(c) Discuss the pathophysiology of this condition *(3 marks)*

(d) What are the indications of surgery in this condition? *(3 marks)*

Question 15

A 5-year-old boy is referred from the school clinic with a persistent hearing loss in one ear. A diagnosis of 'glue ear' is made.

(a) (i) Discuss the nature of the hearing loss *(2 marks)*
(ii) List three predisposing factors *(2 marks)*

(b) Describe the appearance of the eardrum in this condition *(2 marks)*

(c) Discuss two methods of surgically treating this condition *(4 marks)*

6

Endocrinology and Breast

Question 1

A 35-year-old woman presents to the surgical clinic with a gradually enlarging asymptomatic swelling in the front of her neck.

(a) (i) State the differential clinical diagnoses *(2 marks)*

    (ii) How would you clinically distinguish one from the other? *(2 marks)*

(b) Discuss the investigations that you would perform to confirm your clinical impression *(2 marks)*

(c) If you had diagnosed a goitre, state the clinical findings that would require surgical intervention *(4 marks)*

Question 2

A 30-year-old woman presents to the surgical clinic with symptoms of restlessness, insomnia and a preference for cooler weather. She has a pulse rate of 110/min and a painless swelling of her thyroid gland.

(a) (i) State your probable diagnosis   *(1 mark)*

(ii) List other clinical features that would support this diagnosis   *(3 marks)*

(b) State the investigations that you would perform to assess her thyroid function   *(3 marks)*

(c) Discuss the management of this condition   *(3 marks)*

Question 3

A 64-year-old woman presents to the surgical clinic with a long-standing thyroid swelling, complaining of recent onset of pain in the neck and hoarseness.

(a) Write a short note on the clinical findings that would assist you in reaching a diagnosis   *(3 marks)*

(b) State the probable cause of the hoarseness and the examination that you would carry out to confirm this
                    (2 marks;)

(c) (i) State the investigations that you would request to confirm your clinical diagnosis   *(3 marks)*

(ii) What is referred to as a 'cold nodule' on thyroid imaging?   *(2 marks)*

Question 4

A 46-year-old woman in chronic renal failure sustained a pathological fracture of her hip.

(a) Discuss briefly the metabolic basis for the fracture

(3 marks)

(b) Her serum parathyroid hormone (PTH) titres were raised. Explain the parathyroid hyperfunction in relation to renal failure *(3 marks)*

(c) State how you would counteract the elevated PTH titres

(4 marks)

Question 5

A 25-year-old, otherwise healthy, woman gives a 12-month history of headaches of increasing frequency, accompanied by flushes and sweats. Her BP is 180/120 mmHg and a CT scan of her abdomen reveals a right-sided adrenal tumour measuring 5.5 cm. Her 24-hour urinary levels of metanephrines and vanillylmandelic acid were significantly raised.

(a) (i) State the likely diagnosis *(1 mark)*

    (ii) What other biochemical test(s) would confirm your diagnosis? *(2 marks)*

(b) (i) Discuss the functional disorders caused by this lesion *(2 marks)*

    (ii) Give the medical management of these *(3 marks)*

    (iii) State the definitive treatment for this disease

(2 marks)

Question 6

A 58-year-old woman presents with a 9-month history of progressive fatigue, weight gain and spontaneous skin bruising. She was found to be hypertensive, with impaired glucose tolerance.

(a) (i) State the endocrine disorder *(1 mark)*

(ii) Name one laboratory investigation that would confirm your diagnosis *(1 mark)*

(b) (i) State the source of this disease *(1 mark)*

(ii) Give one investigation to define the anatomical site of the lesion *(1 mark)*

(iii) List three other endocrine disorders that may arise from the same gland *(3 marks)*

(c) Discuss the principles of treating this patient *(3 marks)*

Question 7

A worried 46-year-old woman, attending the breast clinic, gives a 3-week history of a blood-stained discharge from her right nipple.

(a) (i) List three possible abnormal findings during your examination of her breast *(2 marks)*

(ii) List other anatomical regions that you would include in your examination *(2 marks)*

(iii) List three clinical diagnoses that you would consider *(3 marks)*

(b) List three specific investigations that would assist you in arriving at a diagnosis *(3 marks)*

Question 8

An anxious 36-year-old woman, attending the breast clinic, gives a 2-week history of an asymptomatic lump in her left breast.

(a) (i) List the clinical characteristics of the presenting
         lesion   *(2 marks)*
     (ii) State the sites of lymphatic drainage of the breast
                                                    (2 marks)

(b) List the investigations that would assist in confirming
     your clinical diagnosis   *(2 marks)*

(c) List the treatment modalities available for breast
     malignancy   *(4 marks)*

Question 9

A 78-year-old woman presents to the breast clinic with an asymptomatic, hard and irregular mobile lump in her right breast.

(a) (i) State the most likely histological diagnosis *(1 mark)*
     (ii) How would you assess distant spread?   *(3 marks)*

(b) The lump has been present for over 6 years with little
     alteration in size:
     (i)   Is the diagnosis of malignancy still likely? *(1 mark)*
     (ii) How would you treat her if malignancy were
           confirmed?   *(2 marks)*
     (iii) If she declines your offer of treatment, what would
           be the likely outcome?   *(3 marks)*

Question 10

A 55-year-old woman is referred to the breast clinic after a screening mammography.

(a) State three investigations that you would perform on a barely palpable, right-sided breast lump   *(3 marks)*

(b) The lump is removed under stereotactic guidance and found to be a lobular carcinoma with vascular invasion. List your investigations for the presence of distant metastases   *(3 marks)*

(c) State the principles of treatment   *(4 marks)*

7

QUESTIONS

Cardiothoracic Surgery

Question 1

An 18-month-old boy presents with episodes of breathlessness and cyanosis, usually after a feed; there is no history of vomiting. On examination bowel sounds are heard over his left chest wall.

(a) (i) State your working diagnosis *(1 mark)*

(ii) List the radiological findings on chest radiograph
(3 marks)

(b) List the complications of delayed diagnosis *(3 marks)*

(c) State the principles of surgical treatment *(3 marks)*

Question 2

A 46-year-old man gives a 4-month history of cough and breathlessness, with right-sided chest pain. He has fever and appears toxic. Clinical examination elicits dullness on percussion and absence of breath sounds on the affected side. Chest radiograph reveals a right-sided effusion. A thoracoscopy is arranged.

(a) What is the diagnosis and how you would manage this condition? *(4 marks)*

(b) Write a short note on thoracoscopy *(3 marks)*

(c) List the aetiological factors associated with this diagnosis *(3 marks)*

Question 3

A 71-year-old woman who is a long-term smoker presents with an enlarged asymptomatic lymph node at the root of her neck.

(a) List four malignant diseases that may present thus *(2 marks)*

(b) Biopsy of the node reveals a deposit of small cell carcinoma. State your clinical diagnosis and the investigations to confirm this *(4 marks)*

(c) State the principles of surgical treatment of this lesion *(4 marks)*

Question 4

A 58-year-old man who has smoked heavily for nearly 30 years was seen in surgical outpatient clinic complaining of chronic cough, dyspnoea and two recent episodes of haemoptysis. He has also lost weight and his chest radiograph shows a 3 cm cavitated lesion in the right upper lobe. You tell this man that he probably has got a neoplastic lesion in his lung.

(a) What are the histological subtypes of the most common type of lung cancer? *(4 marks)*

(b) How will you investigate a patient with a suspected lung cancer? *(3 marks)*

(c) Discuss the role of surgery in the management of lung cancer. *(3 marks)*

Question 5

A 68-year-old man presents in the Emergency Department with a history of progressively increasing shortness of breath of 2-years' duration. He also gives history of chest discomfort, pleuritic pain and easy fatigability over the last 6 months. Further enquiry reveals that he had worked for 35 years in a shipping yard. His chest radiograph reveals nodular thickening of the pleura on both sides with decreased size of the right lung field and ipsilateral small pleural effusion.

(a) What is the most likely diagnosis? *(1 mark)*

(b) Discuss the pathophysiology of this condition? *(3 marks)*

(c) How is this condition diagnosed? *(3 marks)*

(d) Discuss the role of surgery in the management of this condition? *(3 marks)*

Question 6

A 68-year-old man complaining of exertional chest pain was investigated and found to have an aortic stenosis with normal coronary arteries. He is referred for aortic valve replacement.

(a) List three common causes of aortic stenosis   *(3 marks)*

(b) What is the pathophysiology of aortic stenosis?
(2 marks)

(c) What options are available for valve replacement in this patient?   *(2 marks)*

(d) Discuss the pros and cons of different types of prosthetic valves   *(3 marks)*

Question 7

A 69-year old pensioner suffers from angina of effort that had progressively worsened over a 20-month period despite medical measures to control his symptoms.

(a) (i)   State your probable diagnosis   *(1 mark)*

(ii) State two non-invasive investigations to confirm your diagnosis   *(1 mark)*

(iii) What information would be obtained from these investigations?   *(2 marks)*

(b)   Write a note on the radiological method used to investigate and treat this disease   *(3 marks)*

(c) Write a note on the principles of surgical treatment of this disease   *(3 marks)*

Question 8

A 58-year-old diabetic and hypertensive man with exertional angina was investigated and found to have triple-vessel coronary artery disease. He was referred for coronary artery bypass surgery as a result of the severity of his coronary artery disease.

(a) Briefly describe the normal coronary anatomy.

(3 marks)

(b) What conduit options are available for doing coronary artery bypass grafting? *(2 marks)*

(c) What is a cardiopulmonary bypass machine? *(2 marks)*

(d) What are the advantages and disadvantages of performing coronary artery bypass surgery on cardiopulmonary bypass? *(3 marks)*

8

Upper Alimentary Tract

Question 1

A 36-year-old woman with poor oral hygiene complains of a colicky postprandial swelling of the submandibular gland. Her condition is relapsing and remitting in nature.

(a) What is the most likely diagnosis? *(1 mark)*

(b) What simple investigation can confirm your diagnosis? *(2 marks)*

(c) Name three conditions that may be considered in the differential diagnosis *(3 marks)*

(d) What is the pathophysiology of this condition? *(2 marks)*

(e) Outline the management of this condition *(2 marks)*

Question 2

A 40-year-old man presents to the surgical clinic with a 2-year history of an asymptomatic, slow-growing, firm lump on the side of his face just below the lobe of his ear.

(a) (i) State the likely diagnosis *(1 mark)*

   (ii) List the characteristics of the lesion that you would ascertain on examination *(3 marks)*

(b) A request was made for cytological confirmation by percutaneous needle biopsy of the lesion. Give your comments *(2 marks)*

(c) (i) Write a note on the principles of surgical treatment *(3 marks)*

   (ii) What structures must be preserved from injury? *(1 mark)*

Question 3

A 29-year-old man is referred to the Emergency Department with a 10-day history of progressive pain and swelling of the floor of his mouth and upper part of his neck. He was pyrexial, with inflamed palpable nodes in the neck.

(a) (i) State the likely diagnosis and the anatomical planes involved in the inflammatory process *(2 marks)*

   (ii) List the pathogenic organisms that are associated with this lesion *(2 marks)*

(b) (i) What are the consequences if left untreated? *(2 marks)*

   (ii) How would you treat this lesion? *(4 marks)*

Question 4

A 76-year-old man complains of a sore tongue. On examination a 1-cm ulcer was present on the posterolateral aspect of the tongue with a patchy, white, hyperkeratotic discoloration of the surrounding mucosa.

(a) List the clinical findings that would suggest a malignant ulcer *(3 marks)*

(b) What is the surrounding mucosal lesion called? List the aetiological factors associated with this lesion
(3 marks)

(c) The ulcer on the tongue was found to be a squamous carcinoma. Discuss the principles of treatment
(4 marks)

Question 5

A newborn baby is found to regurgitate his feeds and has developed a post-aspiration respiratory infection.

(a) (i) State your working diagnosis *(1 mark)*
    (ii) State the radiological investigation required to confirm your diagnosis *(1 mark)*

(b) (i) Write a note or illustrate the congenital malformations that may present thus *(4 marks)*
    (ii) State a simple procedure that could be performed at birth to exclude this abnormality *(2 marks)*

(c) What are the principles of treatment? *(2 marks)*

Question 6

A 45-year-old woman with complaints of dysphagia and regurgitation on lying down had a barium swallow, which showed a dilated oesophagus with slow passage of contrast into the stomach. The distal oesophagus was narrowed and had a bird's beak appearance.

(a) What is the most likely diagnosis? *(1 mark)*

(b) What are the usual clinical features of this condition? *(3 marks)*

(c) How will you investigate such a patient? *(3 marks)*

(d) Discuss the management of such a patient *(3 marks)*

Question 7

A 71-year-old man is referred to the surgical clinic with increasing difficulty in swallowing and significant weight loss over a period of 6 months.

(a) What other aspects of the history would assist you in arriving at a clinical diagnosis? *(2 marks)*

(b) (i) List the possible causes of dysphagia in this patient *(3 marks)*

(ii) Name two investigations that would confirm your clinical diagnosis. What information would you obtain from each? *(2 marks)*

(c) Write a note on the aetiological factors associated with any two diagnoses *(3 marks)*

Question 8

A 34-year-old, otherwise healthy, woman gives a history of heartburn and belching with waterbrash.

(a) (i) State your probable diagnosis *(1 mark)*

(ii) Write a short note on the underlying lesion *(3 marks)*

(iii) State one investigation that you would perform to confirm your diagnosis *(1 mark)*

(b) (i) Discuss briefly the measures that you would advise to alleviate her symptoms *(2 marks)*

(ii) State the surgical procedures that would effect a cure *(3 marks)*

Question 9

A 4-month-old infant is referred with a history of projectile vomiting and poor weight gain since birth. His mother had felt a lump in his abdomen after feeds.

(a) (i) State your working diagnosis *(2 marks)*

(ii) List two differential diagnoses *(2 marks)*

(iii) What is the nature of the lump that the mother felt? *(1 mark)*

(b) Write a short note on the pathophysiology of this lesion *(2 marks)*

(c) Discuss the principles of treatment *(3 marks)*

Question 10

A 40-year-old male business executive presents with a 6-month history of upper abdominal pain that comes on in the evenings and wakes him in the early hours of the morning. Symptoms are relieved by food, milk and antacids.

(a) (i) State your clinical diagnosis *(1 mark)*

(ii) Discuss briefly the aetiological factors associated with this disease *(2 marks)*

(b) State one investigation that would demonstrate both the site and the appearance of the lesion, and write a note on how this investigation is performed *(2 marks)*

(c) (i) Discuss briefly the principles of treating this disease *(3 marks)*

(ii) List the complications of this disease *(2 marks)*

Question 11

A 39-year-old man with a 6-month history of dyspepsia unresponsive to antacids is found to have an apparently normal gastric mucosa on endoscopy.

(a) List the tests that you would perform on antral mucosal biopsies obtained in order to reach a diagnosis

(3 marks)

(b) (i) If a bacterial presence was detected, state the probable diagnosis *(1 mark)*

(ii) How would you treat this infection? *(3 marks)*

(c) Write a note on the association of this pathogen with lesions of the stomach and duodenum *(3 marks)*

Question 12

A 36-year-old woman on anti-inflammatory medication for symptoms of rheumatoid arthritis developed severe upper abdominal pain of sudden onset. She is found to be pyrexial with a rigid abdomen.

(a) (i) State the probable diagnosis *(2 marks)*

(ii) List the radiological features to confirm your diagnosis *(2 marks)*

(b) Write a note on your treatment measures, including surgical measures if appropriate *(4 marks)*

(c) State your measures to prevent recurrence of this disease *(2 marks)*

Question 13

A 43-year-old man gives a 4-month history of dyspepsia, abdominal distension and weight loss. He is of pallid complexion with negative abdominal findings; however, a lymph node was palpable in the left supraventricular fossa.

(a) State the significance of the enlarged node and how it would assist in arriving at a diagnosis *(2 marks)*

(b) List three investigations that you would perform *(3 marks)*

(c) State three types of gastric cancer and outline the principles of treatment *(5 marks)*

Question 14

A 38-year-old man presents to the Emergency Department vomiting blood. An emergency upper gastrointestinal endoscopy reveals bleeding from oesophageal varices.

(a) How would you control the bleeding? *(4 marks)*

(b) State the pathophysiology of this condition *(3 marks)*

(c) What would be your follow-up protocol for this patient? *(3 marks)*

Question 15

A 32-year-old man underwent an elective splenectomy for hypersplenism.

(a) List the three main types of postoperative bleeding in this patient *(3 marks)*

(b) How would you manage such a haemorrhage in the immediate postoperative period? *(4 marks)*

(c) State the factors that may increase his susceptibility to infections, and your preventive measures *(3 marks)*

9

Liver, Gallbladder and Pancreas

Question 1

A 16-year-old boy, a recent visitor to this country, is found to be moderately pale and febrile, and to have a large and tender spleen.

(a) List six causes of a chronically enlarged spleen

(3 marks)

(b) What do you understand by the term 'hypersplenism'?

(3 marks)

(c) Outline the indications for splenectomy in this patient

(4 marks)

Question 2

A 40-year-old housewife complains of severe right upper abdominal pain radiating to the back, 2 hours after eating fried food.

(a) (i) Give your working diagnosis *(1 mark)*

(ii) Give three physical signs that you would expect to support this diagnosis *(2 marks)*

(iii) Give one non-invasive investigation to support your diagnosis *(1 mark)*

(b) Write a note on the pathogenesis of the disease *(3 marks)*

(c) Discuss briefly the principles of surgical treatment *(3 marks)*

Question 3

A 66-year-old woman with a history of calculus cholecystitis is admitted as an emergency feeling acutely ill, with progressive jaundice, right upper quadrant pain and rigors over the previous 3 days.

(a) (i) State your probable diagnosis *(1 mark)*

(ii) Outline the causation and pathogenesis of this condition *(2 marks)*

(iii) State the immediate blood investigations that you would request, giving the reason for each *(3 marks)*

(b) State two non-invasive methods of visualising the biliary tree in order to confirm your diagnosis *(1 mark)*

(c) Discuss the principles of treatment *(3 marks)*

Question 4

A 34-year-old woman complains of increasing pain and becomes progressively jaundiced soon after an elective cholecystectomy.

(a) (i) State the most likely cause of her jaundice *(1 mark)*

(ii) State an invasive investigation that would confirm your diagnosis *(1 mark)*

(iii) How would you prepare the patient for this procedure? *(2 marks)*

(b) She develops a tender abdomen with rebound, rigors and a raised WBC. State your diagnosis *(2 marks)*

(c) Write a note on the measures that the surgeon should adopt to avoid these complications *(4 marks)*

Question 5

A 38-year-old woman presents acutely with symptoms of small bowel obstruction. She gave a 6-month history of fatty food intolerance and upper right-sided abdominal pain with mild episodes of jaundice.

(a) (i) State the likely diagnosis *(1 mark)*

(ii) What is the pathogenesis of the disease? *(1 mark)*

(iii) List the salient features on the abdominal radiograph *(2 marks)*

(b) How would you treat her bowel obstruction? *(3 marks)*

(c) Write a short note on your management of the underlying pathology *(3 marks)*

Question 6

A 48-year-old woman with a history of gallstones presents with severe upper abdominal pain and vomiting. On examination, her abdomen is rigid and tender with absent bowel sounds. An erect abdominal radiograph was normal. Both serum amylase titres and WBC were raised.

(a) (i) State the probable diagnosis   *(1 mark)*

    (ii) Give two main causes for this condition   *(2 marks)*

(b) Outline your management   *(4 marks)*

(c) List the complications of this disease   *(3 marks)*

Question 7

A 78-year-old man gives a 6-week history of progressive jaundice, anorexia and weight loss. Clinically, he is malnourished and pale, and abdominal examination revealed a palpable gallbladder and a liver edge.

(a) State the probable diagnosis and list the investigations that you would require to confirm it   *(3 marks)*

(b) (i) List your treatment options for this patient

        (3 marks)

    (ii) What factors would decide against major curative surgery?   *(2 marks)*

(c) If the patient underwent an abdominal operation, list the postoperative complications that are associated with jaundice   *(2 marks)*

Question 8

A 15-year-old boy sustained blunt injury to the upper abdomen in a cycling accident; he underwent surgical repair of a laceration to the right lobe of the liver and drainage of the abdomen.

(a) Postoperatively he vomits fresh blood:

    (i) State two possible causative factors   *(1 mark)*

    (ii) How would you treat these complications?

                                         (4 marks)

(b) The abdominal drain drains a clear fluid with a high amylase content:

    (i) State the significance of this finding   *(1 mark)*

    (ii) How would you identify the lesion?   *(2 marks)*

(c) The abdominal drain drains bile instead:

    (i) State the probable lesion   *(1 mark)*

    (ii) How would you define the lesion?   *(1 mark)*

Question 9

A 30-year-old man presents to the Emergency Department complaining of severe central abdominal pain and nausea of 7 days' duration.

(a) In the absence of significant clinical findings a working diagnosis of acute non-specific abdominal pain was made:

   (i) What do you understand by this statement?

   (1 mark)

   (ii) Give examples of psychosomatic states that may be associated with this presentation   *(2 marks)*

(b) Further enquiries revealed a history of alcoholism, with previous similar clinical presentations:

   (i) State the probable diagnosis and the investigations required to confirm this   *(3 marks)*

   (ii) Write a note on the principles of treatment

   (4 marks)

Small and Large Bowel

Question 1

A neonate presents at birth with a defect in the abdominal wall, covered by a transparent sac containing loops of intestine. The umbilical cord was attached at its apex.

(a) (i) What is this condition called? *(1 mark)*

    (ii) Write a note on the development of this anomaly *(3 marks)*

(b) Write a note on the principles of treatment for this condition *(3 marks)*

(c) List three malformations of the alimentary tract resulting in failure of canalisation of the lumen *(3 marks)*

Question 2

A 2-week-old pre-term baby weighing 1500 g developed abdominal distension, circulatory collapse and bloody stools upon commencement of enteral feeding.

(a) What is the likely diagnosis? *(1 mark)*

(b) What is the aetiology of this condition? *(3 marks)*

(c) What is the mainstay of diagnostic imaging in this condition? *(1 mark)*

(d) List findings on an abdominal radiograph in this condition *(2 marks)*

(e) Discuss briefly the management of this condition *(3 marks)*

Question 3

A 77-year-old woman is referred to the surgical clinic with a 3-month history of alteration in bowel habit, with intermittent passage of loose motions containing mucus and blood.

(a) List the possible causes of her symptoms *(3 marks)*

(b) If dietary and infective causes are excluded, outline the specific measures that you would adopt to arrive at a diagnosis *(4 marks)*

(c) If abdominal examination revealed hepatomegaly and ascites, state the further investigations that you would request and the information obtained therefrom *(3 marks)*

Question 4

A 42-year-old healthy woman with no previous medical history is seen in the Emergency Department after a complaint of pain in her right flank. She was noticed to have cystic collections of gas localised to the wall of the colon on a plain abdominal radiograph.

(a) What is the condition seen on plain abdominal radiograph? *(1 mark)*

(b) List three causes for this radiological finding *(3 marks)*

(c) What is the significance of this radiological finding? *(2 marks)*

(d) What is the management of this condition? *(3 marks)*

(e) What is the prognosis of this condition? *(1 mark)*

Question 5

A 3-month-old infant is referred to the Emergency Department with a 3-day history of fretfulness and colic. He had vomited bile-stained fluid the previous day and passed blood-stained mucus per rectum.

(a) (i) State the likely diagnosis *(1 mark)*

(ii) Write a note on the factors that may be associated with this condition *(2 marks)*

(b) What would be the findings on abdominal examination? *(3 marks)*

(c) (i) State one investigation that is used both to confirm the diagnosis and to treat the condition *(1 mark)*

(ii) How is this procedure performed? *(3 marks)*

Question 6

A 45-year-old, 70 kg man is admitted with symptoms of acute small bowel obstruction.

(a) List the findings on abdominal radiograph that would confirm the diagnosis *(2 marks)*

(b) (i) How would you assess the accompanying fluid and electrolyte derangement? *(3 marks)*

 (ii) How would you treat it? *(3 marks)*

(c) If the obstruction results from adhesions as a consequence of previous abdominal surgery, state your management *(2 marks)*

Question 7

A 4-day-old neonate is seen in the Emergency Department with progressive abdominal distension and not passing meconium since birth.

(a) List the causes of large bowel obstruction in the newborn *(2 marks)*

(b) Rectal examination on this patient was followed by spontaneous passage of a large quantity of meconium:
 (i) State the probable diagnosis *(1 mark)*
 (ii) Write a note on its pathogenesis *(3 marks)*

(c) (i) State two investigations to confirm your diagnosis *(2 marks)*
 (ii) State the principles of surgical treatment *(2 marks)*

Question 8

A 59-year-old woman is admitted with a 3-week history of progressively severe crampy lower abdominal pain and distension. She has not opened her bowels for the past 9 days, feels nauseous and has vomited twice over the previous 2 days.

(a) (i) State your expected clinical findings   *(2 marks)*

     (ii) What is your working diagnosis?   *(1 mark)*

(b) (i) State one radiological investigation that would confirm your diagnosis   *(1 mark)*

     (ii) List the findings   *(2 marks)*

(c) State your initial management of this patient   *(4 marks)*

Question 9

An otherwise healthy 44-year-old woman gives a history of many years of increasing constipation that followed a difficult pregnancy and confinement. She is currently dependent on laxatives.

(a) List two causative factors   *(2 marks)*

(b) How would you assist this patient's symptoms?   *(3 marks)*

(c) Outline your management   *(5 marks)*

Question 10

A 61-year-old man known to have diverticular disease on a previous colonoscopy is admitted as an emergency with crampy lower abdominal pains, fever, malaise and anorexia. Abdominal examination reveals mild peritonism in the lower left quadrant.

(a) State the probable cause of his symptoms   *(2 marks)*

(b) List two investigations that would support your diagnosis   *(4 marks)*

(c) Outline your management   *(4 marks)*

Question 11

A 35-year-old man is referred to the surgical clinic with a 4-month history of painless rectal bleeding after defecation.

(a) (i) How would you examine the anorectum to arrive at a diagnosis?   *(3 marks)*

   (ii) List three diseases of the colon that may present thus   *(3 marks)*

(b) The patient also complains of an intermittent fleshy protrusion at the anus:

   (i) State the most likely cause   *(1 mark)*

   (ii) List three procedures used to treat this condition *(3 marks)*

Question 12

A 79-year-old woman with a vague history of intermittent crampy lower abdominal pains underwent a colonoscopic examination. A cluster of polyps covering a 7 cm segment was seen in the descending colon.

(a) List three histological varieties of benign colonic polyps *(2 marks)*

(b) How would you manage this condition? *(5 marks)*

(c) Outline the aetiology of this condition *(3 marks)*

Question 13

A 68-year-old woman presents with a 6-week history of tenesmus and the passage of blood-stained mucus in her motions. Examination reveals an ulcerating lesion in the rectum.

(a) (i) How would you characterise the clinical features of this lesion? *(3 marks)*

(ii) State one investigation that is required to make a definitive diagnosis *(2 marks)*

(b) A diagnosis of a rectal adenocarcinoma is made:

(i) State the most frequent site of blood-borne metastases *(1 mark)*

(ii) What is your method for its detection? *(1 mark)*

(iii) Write a note on the surgical treatment of this lesion *(3 marks)*

Question 14

A 43-year-old manual worker presented to the Emergency Department with a 4-day history of fever and a painful, tender, fluctuant swelling immediately lateral to the anus.

(a) (i) State the probable diagnosis *(1 mark)*

(ii) Write a note on the evolution of this lesion
(3 marks)

(b) He was sent home on a course of antibiotics. Soon afterwards the swelling ruptured draining pus, and the pain and temperature settled. However, the wound continued to discharge intermittently over the next 3 months:

(i) State the complication that had ensued *(1 mark)*

(ii) How should his original lesion have been treated?
(2 marks)

(iii) Write a note on the principles of treating the current complication *(3 marks)*

11

Urology

Question 1

A 5-year-old boy presents to the paediatric surgical clinic with an incidental discovery by his mother of a left flank mass.

(a) (i) List four lesions of the kidney that may present thus *(2 marks)*

(ii) State three imaging procedures used to arrive at a diagnosis *(3 marks)*

(b) If these investigations reveal a malignant tumour of the left kidney:

(i) State three investigations required to determine the presence of distant metastases *(2 marks)*

(ii) Outline the three modalities of treatment *(3 marks)*

Question 2

A 35-year-old man in end-stage renal failure underwent cadaveric renal transplantation. Postoperatively he remains oliguric.

(a) List four possible causes for the oliguria (*2 marks*)

(b) Write a note of the investigations that you would perform to arrive at a diagnosis (*3 marks*)

(c) (i) List the drugs used for immunosuppression after a transplantation (*2 marks*)

(ii) Write a note on the complications associated with their use (*3 marks*)

Question 3

A 70-year-old man complains of passing bubbles of gas in his urine. Six months previously he had undergone surgical removal of a colonic tumour, followed by radiotherapy to the region.

(a) (i) What is this symptom called? (*1 mark*)

(ii) State two probable causes for this symptom (*2 marks*)

(b) List the investigations that would confirm your diagnosis (*3 marks*)

(c) List four other diseases that may produce this complication (*4 marks*)

Question 4

A 28-year-old woman is referred to the urology clinic with a 3-month history of severe intermittent unilateral loin pain radiating to the groin, accompanied by nausea and vomiting.

(a) (i) State your clinical diagnosis   *(1 mark)*

      (ii) What immediate investigation would confirm your diagnosis at the bedside?   *(2 marks)*

(b) Outline your management   *(5 marks)*

(c) List four predisposing causes   *(2 marks)*

Question 5

A 10-year-old Asian boy presents as an emergency in acute urinary retention. He gives a history of frequency with episodes of strangury, penile tip pain and haematuria over the past 18 months.

(a) State your working diagnosis   *(2 marks)*

(b) Outline your investigations   *(4 marks)*

(c) How would you treat this condition?   *(4 marks)*

Question 6

A middle-aged man is seen in the surgical clinic with an asymptomatic intermittent swelling in his right groin. He gives a 12-month history of nocturnal frequency and dribbling.

(a) State the nature of his groin swelling and examination findings that would support your diagnosis *(3 marks)*

(b) State the probable cause of his urinary symptoms and discuss the relevant findings on examination *(3 marks)*

(c) Discuss briefly the management of this patient
(4 marks)

Question 7

A 75-year-old man is returned to the ward after a transurethral prostatectomy. He complains of severe suprapubic pain and becomes hypotensive.

(a) State two surgical complications that would present thus *(4 marks)*

(b) State two causes of prostatic enlargement that may require prostatectomy *(2 marks)*

(c) List the complications that may arise if symptoms of prostatism are left untreated *(4 marks)*

Question 8

A 29-year-old man is referred to the surgical clinic with a 6-week history of an asymptomatic swelling in the right side of his scrotum.

(a) (i) State the structures that may be involved *(3 marks)*

(ii) Describe how you would, by examination, localise the lesion *(2 marks)*

(b) (i) List three testicular tumours found in young adults *(3 marks)*

(ii) State the principles of treating testicular tumours *(2 marks)*

Question 9

A 15-year-old boy presents to the Emergency Department with sudden onset of severe pain in his left testicle 2 hours earlier.

(a) (i) State the likely diagnosis *(1 mark)*

(ii) State your findings in support of the diagnosis *(3 marks)*

(b) Write a short note on your treatment *(3 marks)*

(c) If the patient presented 48 h after the onset of symptoms, how would this alter your management? *(3 marks)*

Question 10

A 28-year-old man is referred to the urology clinic complaining of impotence.

(a) State three causes for this *(3 marks)*

(b) Seminal fluid analysis suggested sterility. On what criteria would this report be based? *(3 marks)*

(c) (i) State a chronic infection that may produce sterility in this patient *(1 mark)*

(ii) How would you confirm your diagnosis? *(3 marks)*

Question 11

A 34-year-old, otherwise healthy, man presents with progressive symptoms of straining to void, with poor urinary stream and dribbling. An indurated area was palpable in the line of the penile urethra.

(a) State the probable diagnosis and list the probable causes of this condition *(3 marks)*

(b) State the complications of this lesion *(3 marks)*

(c) Write a note on the principles of treatment *(4 marks)*

Question 12

A 2-year-old toddler is referred to the surgical clinic with a history from the parents of irritation and ballooning of the foreskin during micturition over a 4-month period.

(a) (i) State the probable diagnosis   *(2 marks)*
        (ii) How would you confirm your diagnosis? *(2 marks)*

(b) What are the complications of this condition? *(3 marks)*

(c) State your treatment   *(3 marks)*

Question 13

A female neonate is found at birth to have a 5 cm defect in the lower abdominal wall through which there is extravasation of urine.

(a) State your diagnosis   *(2 marks)*

(b) List the structures that may be visible through the defect   *(3 marks)*

(c) State the associated anomalies that may be present
                                                       (2 marks)

(d) How would you manage this condition?   *(3 marks)*

Question 14

A 35-year-old woman was seen in the urology outpatient clinic six months after childbirth complaining of loss of small amounts of urine with coughing, laughing, sneezing, or exercising. She was told by the consultant that she has stress incontinence.

(a) Define stress incontinence of urine and discuss its causes in a 35-year-old woman   (3 marks)

(b) How would you investigate her symptoms?   *(3 marks)*

(c) State the principles of treatment   *(4 marks)*

12

Vascular Surgery

Question 1

A 79-year-old man presents to the Emergency Department with a 4-hour history of sudden onset of severe pain and numbness in his left leg extending up to his mid-thigh.

(a) State your working diagnosis and the predisposing vascular diseases *(3 marks)*

(b) List the clinical findings in the limb supporting your diagnosis *(3 marks)*

(c) Write a note on the treatment *(4 marks)*

Question 2

A 68-year-old man complains of gradual onset of right calf claudication radiating up to his thigh on walking distances exceeding 75 metres.

(a) (i) State your likely diagnosis and the anatomical site(s) of his lesion *(2 marks)*

(ii) Write a short note on the disease process causing his symptoms *(3 marks)*

(b) Give four common risk factors in this disease *(2 marks)*

(c) What measures would you advise him to adopt to alleviate his symptoms, to stop progression of the disease and to improve his walking distance? *(3 marks)*

Question 3

A 59-year-old woman complains of rest pain in her left foot, keeping her awake at night. She also has difficulty in walking.

(a) List the clinical findings that would lead to a working diagnosis *(4 marks)*

(b) (i) Name one radiological investigation that you would request to demonstrate the lesion *(1 mark)*

(ii) Write a short note on how radiological procedures may be used to treat her symptoms *(2 marks)*

(c) Discuss briefly the surgical options available to relieve her symptoms *(3 marks)*

Question 4

A 68-year-old man underwent a femoral arteriogram and balloon angioplasty for an external iliac arterial stenosis.

(a) List the symptoms and clinical findings that would have led to this procedure *(3 marks)*

(b) Soon afterwards he complained of severe pain in the limb, which had become blanched and pulseless:

(i) State two likely causes for this complication *(2 marks)*

(ii) State your management *(3 marks)*

(c) List the risk factors in the development of peripheral vascular disease *(2 marks)*

Question 5

A 76-year-old man presents with a pulsatile swelling in his right groin 3 days after a coronary angioplasty at the site where the cardiac catheter was introduced.

(a) (i) State the most likely diagnosis *(1 mark)*

(ii) State one non-invasive investigation for confirmation *(1 mark)*

(iii) How would you treat this? *(2 marks)*

(b) The patient developed a cold, painful and pulseless lower limb immediately after the coronary angioplasty:

(i) State two probable causes *(2 marks)*

(ii) How would you treat each of these complications? *(4 marks)*

Question 6

A 75-year-old man is referred to the surgical clinic with an incidental finding of a palpable, pulsatile and expansile upper abdominal mass of approximately 10 cm in diameter.

(a) (i) State the likely diagnosis *(1 mark)*

(ii) Discuss the pathological changes that produced this lesion *(2 marks)*

(b) State one non-invasive investigation that you would request to identify the anatomical limits of the lesion *(1 mark)*

(c) (i) Write short notes on the principles of surgical treatment of this patient *(3 marks)*

(ii) Write short notes on the preoperative preparation of the patient *(3 marks)*

Question 7

A 64-year-old man is admitted to the Emergency Department complaining of severe back pain, radiating to the left loin, accompanied by nausea and feeling faint. He was found to be hypotensive, with a rapid, thready pulse.

(a) (i) State your clinical diagnosis *(1 mark)*

(ii) Outline your resuscitatory measures *(3 marks)*

(b) State the surgical treatment for this condition *(1 mark)*

(c) (i) If he were on long-term warfarin therapy for atrial fibrillation and his INR (international normalised ratio) was found to be > 4.0, what would be your diagnosis? *(2 marks)*

(ii) State your specific treatment measures *(3 marks)*

Question 8

A 70-year-old chronic smoker gives a history of dizzy spells over an 8-month period. More recently he experienced occasional blurring of vision, with transient loss of vision in his right eye.

(a) (i) Give the probable cause of his symptoms *(1 mark)*

(ii) State the underlying factors that may be causative or associated with his disease *(2 marks)*

(b) (i) Name one invasive investigation to confirm your diagnosis *(1 mark)*

(ii) What information would you obtain therefrom? *(2 marks)*

(c) Write a note on your proposed treatment *(4 marks)*

Question 9

A 50-year-old woman with a long history of progressively symptomatic lower limb varicosities bled profusely from a chronic leg ulcer. She presents to the Emergency Department with a tourniquet applied to control the haemorrhage.

(a) Write a note on the pathogenesis of the ulcer and the bleeding therefrom *(3 marks)*

(b) Comment on the method used for haemostasis and state how you would control the bleeding *(3 marks)*

(c) Discuss her management once haemostasis has been achieved *(4 marks)*

Question 10

A middle-aged woman is seen in the surgical clinic with a long history of a painful ulcer over the medial aspect of her left ankle, with swelling of the foot. She also complained of long-standing varicose veins in that limb.

(a) (i) State the type of ulcer and its cause *(1 mark)*

(ii) Comment on the characteristics of the lesion and the state of the surrounding skin *(2 marks)*

(b) (i) Write a short note on the measures that you would adopt to bring about the healing of the ulcer *(2 marks)*

(ii) How would you prevent its recurrence? *(1 mark)*

(c) State two other types of chronic leg ulcers and discuss their pathophysiology *(4 marks)*

Question 11

A 46-year-old woman who had undergone abdominal surgery 5 days earlier develops pain and cramps in her left calf and lower thigh.

(a) Discuss the clinical findings that you would elicit in order to arrive at a diagnosis *(3 marks)*

(b) (i) State a diagnosis that carries potentially lethal complications *(1 mark)*

(ii) Write a short note on the pathophysiology of this condition and its complications *(3 marks)*

(c) Write a short note on the management of this patient *(3 marks)*

Question 12

A 35-year-old woman who had been discharged from hospital 2 days earlier, after abdominal surgery, develops sudden chest pain, with shortness of breath.

(a) (i) What is the most likely diagnosis? *(1 mark)*

(ii) State the two most important investigations to confirm your diagnosis *(2 marks)*

(b) Discuss the treatment for this condition *(5 marks)*

(c) List the preventive measures to avoid this complication *(2 marks)*

QUESTIONS

ICU & Anaesthesia

Question 1

A 62-year-old male patient was admitted to ICU following abdominoperineal resection for a carcinoma involving the anus. On second postoperative day he became increasingly confused and agitated.

(a) List four causes of confusion in ICU   *(4 marks)*

(b) Briefly discuss evaluation of a confused patient
(3 marks)

(c) Briefly outline treatment of a confused patient in ICU
(3 marks)

Question 2

A 52-year-old patient with polytrauma in ICU with no previous history of ulcer peptic disease develops a massive haematemesis and malena on day 7.

(a) What is medical term for this condition?   *(1 mark)*

(b) What causes this condition?   *(2 marks)*

(c) What are the risk factors for this condition in ICU patients?   *(3 marks)*

(d) What prophylactic options are available for this condition?   *(2 marks)*

(e) What complications are associated with the treatment options for this condition?   *(2 marks)*

Question 3

A long-term patient in the ICU needs insertion of a central venous catheter (CVC) for total parenteral nutrition.

(a) What sites are suitable for insertion of a CVC?

(3 marks)

(b) What preparation is needed for insertion and maintenance of a CVC? *(2 marks)*

(c) What precautions are essential in management of a CVC? *(2 marks)*

(d) List three complications associated with CVC insertion? *(3 marks)*

Question 4

A 46-year-old woman is transferred to ICU in shock. The consultant intensivist decides to float a Swan-Ganz catheter to guide the management of this patient.

(a) What is a Swan-Ganz catheter? *(2 marks)*

(b) How is a Swan-Ganz catheter inserted? *(3 marks)*

(c) What information can be obtained by using a Swan-Ganz catheter? *(3 marks)*

(d) List two complications associated with insertion of Swan-Ganz catheter. *(2 marks)*

Question 5

A 63-year-old diabetic is admitted to ICU in septic shock due to uncontrolled sepsis resulting from a carbuncle on the nape of his neck.

(a)   What is sepsis?   *(1 mark)*

(b)   What is systemic inflammatory response syndrome (SIRS)?   *(2 marks)*

(c)   List three conditions other than sepsis that can cause SIRS.   *(3 marks)*

(d)   What is severe sepsis?   *(1 mark)*

(e)   Briefly discuss pathophysiology of sepsis.   *(3 marks)*

Question 6

A 33-year-old man was noticed by the anaesthetist to develop increased muscular rigidity, increased oxygen consumption, increased carbon dioxide production, tachycardia and an increase in body temperature almost an hour after he received general anaesthesia for exploratory laparotomy.

(a)   What is the most likely complication developed by this patient?   *(1 mark)*

(b)   What is the aetiology of this complication?   *(2 marks)*

(c)   What is the pathophysiology of this complication?
                                                       (3 marks)

(d)   Outline the treatment for this complication.
                                                       (4 marks)

Question 7

A 23-year-old trauma victim is brought to the Emergency Department with a flail chest. It was decided to intubate and ventilate the patient using rapid sequence intubation (RSI).

(a) What are indications for an endotracheal intubation?

(3 marks)

(b) What are the contraindications for endotracheal intubation? *(2 marks)*

(c) List three complications of endotracheal intubation.

(3 marks)

(d) What is rapid sequence intubation? *(2 marks)*

Question 8

A 46-year-old man underwent a surgical procedure on his right upper limb under intravenous regional anaestheia and application of a tourniquet.

(a) What physiological changes occur during inflation of tourniquet? *(3 marks)*

(b) What physiological changes occur during deflation of a tourniquet? *(3 marks)*

(c) What are advantages of using a tourniquet? *(2 marks)*

(d) List the complications of using a tourniquet *(2 marks)*

Question 9

A 26-year-old man returned to HDU following a thoracotomy with an epidural catheter.

(a) Enumerate the indications for epidural technique

(4 marks)

(b) Enumerate the contraindications for this technique

(3marks)

(c) Enumerate three complications of this technique

(3 marks)

Question 10

A 45-year-old woman after open cholecystectomy requiring admission to HDU develops troublesome nausea and vomiting.

(a) List two causes for postoperative nausea and vomiting

(2 marks)

(b) Enumerate two complications of postoperative vomiting

(2 marks)

(c) Discuss the pathophysiology of postoperative nausea and vomiting

(3 marks)

(d) Outline the management of postoperative nausea and vomiting

(3 marks)

PART TWO

SAQ Model Answers and Comments

Surgical Physiology

Answer 1

(a) Conjugated bilirubin and alkaline phosphatase are markedly raised (normal: 7 mol/l and 0–306 units/l, respectively); the raised aminotransferases and gamma-glutamyltransferase suggest significant liver damage, which is reflected by a low serum albumin (normal: 25–35 g/l) and decreased plasma prothrombin index   *(4 marks)*

(b) Improve general nutritional status by high protein–calorie diet
Correct hypochromic anaemic
Vitamin K therapy to improve clotting profile   *(3 marks)*

(c) Surgical bleeding (intra- and postoperative)
Poor wound healing
Postoperative liver failure   *(3 marks)*

Comments
Patients in liver failure tolerate anaesthesia or surgery poorly. Child's grading of liver failure in assessing preoperative fitness is based on the serum bilirubin and albumin, presence of ascites, and neurological and nutritional status. Liver failure in the postoperative period requires monitoring and correction of blood sugar and electrolyte abnormalities, namely hypoglycaemia and hypernatraemia. Associated renal failure with hyperkalaemia and uraemia requires dialysis. Postoperative bleeding and infection are

treated with the judicious use of blood products and parenteral antibiotics.

Answer 2

(a) FEV_1/FVC is $2.2/4.2 = 52\%$ and indicates obstructive disease; after the administration of bronchodilators, a persisting low ratio suggests chronic obstructive pulmonary disease (COPD) and an improved ratio suggests chronic asthma *(4 marks)*

(b) Breathing exercises, postural physiotherapy to expectorate secretions
Antibiotics to treat residual infection
Oxygen therapy to improve gaseous exchange
Stop smoking (if applicable) *(3 marks)*

(c) Mechanical ventilatory support with arterial blood gases (ABGs) (pulmonary artery wedge pressures if required) and chest radiological monitoring with selective use of sedation, muscle relaxant and antibiotics in a high-dependency or intensive therapy unit *(3 marks)*

Comment

The ratio FEV_1/FVC is normally 75%. A restrictive lung defect reduces both FEV_1 and FVC so that the ratio remains unaltered or may rise slightly, as in fibrosing alveolitis. An obstructive defect causes a relatively larger reduction in FEV_1 so that the ratio falls, as in emphysema, chronic bronchitis and asthma. Preoperative therapy is aimed at improving lung function to the optimum while recognising the limits imposed by end-stage lung disease. Intensive care and ventilatory support must be available after surgery.

Answer 3

(a) (i) Hyperkalaemia and hypernatraemia
Metabolic acidosis with uraemia *(2 marks)*
(ii) Gram-negative septicaemia
Hypovolaemia *(2 marks)*

(b) Rehydration
Intravenous antibiotic therapy
Fluid challenge with judicious use of loop diuretics
Perioperative haemofiltration if above measures fail to improve urinary output

(c) Acute renal failure is a recognised renal complication of surgery and anaesthesia. Management of postoperative acute renal failure includes the following steps:
Check patency of the catheter.
Give sufficient fluid to restore arterial blood pressure and CVP.
If no response to fluid challenge, give 120mg frusemide.
If no response use renal dose of dopamine.
If no response, haemofiltration and dialysis may be necessary as acute tubular necrosis is likely. *(4 marks)*

Comment

Was this patient's renal function normal before his surgical illness? Evidence of a recent assessment of renal function may point to pre-existing renal disease (chronic nephritis) as the underlying cause of the current renal failure. If previous renal function were normal and the present insult not treated promptly, the pre-renal cause would result in acute tubular necrosis. Overwhelming sepsis or disseminated intravascular coagulation results in renal failure and must be treated with haemodialysis or haemofiltration (peritoneal dialysis is contraindicated in view of abdominal sepsis and impending surgery). Haemodialysis results in a rapid correction of metabolic abnormalities, but also produces significant body fluid fluctuations. Haemofiltration produces fewer haemodynamic changes and is preferable in the acutely ill patient perioperatively.

Answer 4

(a) (i)   Thirst; skin turgor; BP (postural drop); serum
            urea and electrolyte (U&E) measurement; urine
            output   *(1 mark)*

 (ii) Physiological or 0.9% saline; 1.8% dextrose or
            3.0% dextrose in 0.9% saline; Hartmann's
            solution; KCl solution (amount in millimoles
            to be carefully titrated against daily or
            twice daily serum levels)   *(2 marks)*

 (iii) Central venous pressure (CVP) monitoring; 3-
            hourly U&E estimation; hourly urine output;
            daily Hb and packed cell volume (PCV)
            estimation; daily weighing of patient   *(2 marks)*

(b) (i)   Hb, PCV, serum albumin, folate, vitamin B_{12}, iron;
            skinfold thickness by use of callipers   *(2 marks)*

 (ii) Daily calorie and nitrogen requirements are
            calculated on the ideal weight for the patient's
            height and body build. Energy requirements vary
            from 1500 to 3000 kcal per day. Parenterally by
            carbohydrate 40% and lipid 60%, nitrogen
            requirement in the form of amino acids is based
            on replacing existing protein depletion and
            ongoing breakdown in wear and tear   *(3 marks)*

Comment

Calories are provided by carbohydrate and fat. They should be in
proportion to the nitrogen intake in the ratio of 150 kcal to 1 g
nitrogen. Administered nitrogen should not be used as an energy
source, because it would perpetuate the state of negative nitrogen
balance. The patient receiving 2000 kcal would require 13 g
nitrogen daily. Vitamins and trace elements are essential as dietary
supplements for normal metabolic function and must be included
in feeding regimens.

Answer 5

(a) (i) Metabolic (hypokalaemic, hyponatraemic, hypochloraemic) alkalosis　　*(1 mark)*

(ii) The fluid regimen did little to correct the Na^+ and K^+ ion loss in vomit and gastric aspirate　　*(3 marks)*

(b) Gastric outlet obstruction leads to loss of water, Na^+, K^+ and H^+. Antidiuretic hormone (ADH) production is stimulated by the hypothalamus. This results in renal tubular reabsorption of Na^+ and K^+ ions at the expense of H^+; this in turn produces an acid urine, thereby exacerbating the metabolic alkalosis　　*(6 marks)*

Comment

The inappropriate production of acid urine in metabolic alkalosis is a result of renal tubular response to dehydration and low serum Na^+ concentrations by reabsorption of Na^+ and excretion of H^+ and K^+ in order to maintain transcellular ionic equilibrium. Counteractive measures should replace Na^+ and K^+ along with water by infusion with 0.9% saline with KCl supplementation. This would gradually reverse the alkalosis with a rise in urinary pH over the ensuing days.

Answer 6

(a) (i) Surgical trauma stimulates ADH production with retention of salt and water　　*(2 marks)*

(ii) He would require no electrolyte supplements. Water requirements would be less than the normal daily requirement of 2–3 litres/day and would be determined by the CVP reading. Dextrose 5% is transfused to keep the CVP at approximately 2–6 cmH_2O　　*(2 marks)*

CHAPTER 1 – ANSWERS

(b) (i)   A normal CVP and BP would ensure good renal perfusion. A postrenal cause must be excluded by ensuring patency of catheter drainage. A low CVP is treated by volume replacement and persistent low BP with pressure support, using intravenous dopamine or dobutamine. The rate of elevation of serum urea and creatinine would indicate the extent of renal malfunction: this is nearly always the result of acute tubular necrosis caused by prolonged hypotension or a coagulopathy. A renal isotope scan would reveal the functional state of each kidney   *(4 marks)*

      (ii)   Renal failure requires haemofiltration or haemodialysis to lower the urea and creatinine and to maintain electrolyte balance   *(2 marks)*

Comment

Acute tubular necrosis is a sequela of major trauma, surgical or otherwise, where there is significant blood loss resulting in renal ischaemia. Cross-clamping the aorta in the vicinity of the renal arteries may also produce a fall in renal perfusion. Large-volume transfusion with stored blood in the perioperative period may produce a coagulopathy, causing acute intravascular coagulation that may lead to renal damage and failure. Acute tubular necrosis usually recovers, and during recovery there is a diuresis, when large quantities of fluid and electrolytes are lost. Careful monitoring and replacement is therefore essential until complete renal function returns.

Answer 7

(a) (i)   Pyrexial reactions are the result of allergens and Gram-negative endotoxins in the donor blood. The skin rash is produced by agglutination of the donor cells in the skin capillaries as a result of incompatibility with the recipient serum   *(2 marks)*

      (ii)   Stop the transfusion immediately; set up a crystalloid infusion to produce a diuresis. Administer an antihistamine and an antipyretic agent as required   *(2 marks)*

(b) (i) Acute liver failure and hepatic coma are rare complications and are precipitated by underlying liver disease. Some clotting factors are inactivated in stored blood, and a coagulopathy, manifesting as acute intravascular coagulation, leads to a bleeding diathesis in the postoperative period

(2 marks)

(ii) In stored blood the plasma K^+ rises to 30–40 mmol/l and produces hyperkalaemia in the recipient. This may be treated by insulin administration with a covering dextrose infusion or by the ingestion of ion exchange resin (calcium resonium). Citrated blood lowers the plasma Ca^{2+} ion concentration in the recipient and it is treated by administration of calcium gluconate or calcium chloride

(4 marks)

Comment

The signs of a mismatched blood transfusion include fever, chills, breathlessness, and pain in the flanks and chest. These may be followed by hypotension, haemorrhagic phenomena and haemoglobinaemia. The last signals renal damage, which is exacerbated by hypotension and acidosis. The initial reactions occur during the first 30 min of the transfusion, and this period must be closely monitored when setting up a blood transfusion.

Answer 8

(a) (i) Lowered platelet count
Lowered vitamin K levels
Raised prothrombin and partial thromboplastin times *(2 marks)*

(ii) Lowered Hb
Lowered WBC (namely, CD4 cells)
Lowered platelet count
Lowered serum albumin (hypoproteinaemia)
Lowered immunoglobulins *(3 marks)*

(b) (i) Plastic apron and non-porous sterile gowns
Visors or goggles
Double gloving
Theatre footwear or shoe covers *(2 marks)*

(ii) Avoid passing instruments 'hand to hand'
Avoid 'sharps' by using cutting diathermy or a
harmonic scalpel for sharp dissection
Scissors with bevelled ends
Blunt needles
Metal or plastic clips for haemostasis
and wound closure *(3 marks)*

Comment

Patients with HIV infection have an increased risk of primary and
secondary haemorrhage and postsurgical bacterial infection.
Wound healing is also delayed as a result of hypoproteinaemia
from cachexia. The grave dangers of accidental inoculation with
tissue fluids from HIV patients during operations should ensure
familiarity with safety measures formulated to protect theatre
personnel.

Answer 9

(a) (i) Metabolic acidosis *(1 mark)*

(ii) Ketoacidosis, lactic acidosis, renal
failure *(2 marks)*

(b) (i) Plasma glucose, U&Es and creatinine *(3 marks)*

(ii) Intravenous 0.9% saline or Hartmann's solution
Intravenous K^+ infusion guided by U&E
estimation
Intravenous insulin on a sliding scale
Intravenous antibiotics – flucloxacillin (or
cefuroxime) and metronidazole
Measure:
4-hourly ABGs
4-hourly U&Es
2-hourly serum K^+ *(4 marks)*

Comment

A variety of organic acids is produced during metabolic activity and their effects are counteracted by expelling CO_2 in the lungs and excreting acidic urine. During metabolic or surgical illness the body is unable to counter the acid load produced, leading to metabolic acidosis. Determination of the base excess and HCO_3^- levels in arterial blood enables effective counter-measures. In addition to the measures stated, 4.8% $NaHCO_3$ intravenous infusion is indicated if the acidosis is intractable or causing cardiac arrhythmias, confusion or drowsiness.

Answer 10

(a) (i)   He has been unable to maintain adequate nutrition as a result of difficulty in swallowing   *(1 mark)*

 (ii)   Moderate-to-severe protein–calorie (energy) malnutrition   *(1 mark)*

 (iii) Visible muscle wasting with reduced muscle strength. Lax subcutaneous tissue from loss of fat deposits as shown by decreased skinfold thickness   *(2 marks)*

(b) (i)   By either enteral feeding through a fine-bore nasogastric tube percutaneous endoscopic gastrostomy or total parenteral nutrition. By either route 1.5–2.5 litres fluid containing 2000–2500 kcal and 1.5 g protein/kg body weight is infused every 24 hours   *(3 marks)*

 (ii)   Daily measurements of body weight
Input and output fluid charts
Serum U&Es, albumin, glucose and urinary glucose
Twice-weekly measurements of Hb, Ca^{2+}, Mg^{2+}, triglycerides, urinary creatinine, Na^+ and K^+ *(3 marks)*

Comment

Nutrient solutions, whether enteral or parenteral, must be administered in moderate increments during the first 48 hours to avoid hyperosmolarity of the body fluids and to give time for pancreatic adaptation. Extraneous insulin may be required to maintain the blood sugar within normal limits. Vitamins and trace elements are added daily. Skin callipers are used in some centres to quantify subcutaneous fat loss. A feeding gastrostomy or jejunostomy should be avoided if the patient is to undergo surgery for his stricture.

Answer 11

(a) Location of wound
Wound contamination
Presence of foreign bodies   *(3 marks)*

(b) Nutrition
Hormones such as glucocorticoids
Circulatory status   *(3 marks)*

(c) Complications in wound healing can arise from abnormalities in any of the basic components of the repair process. These aberrations can be grouped into three general categories:
(i)   *Deficient scar formation*:
      – wound dehiscence
      – ulceration
(ii) *Excessive formation of the repair components*:
      – hypertrophic scar
      – keloid
      – exuberant granulation
      – desmoids or aggressive fibromatoses
(iii) *Formation of contractures*   *(4 marks)*

Comment

The healing wound is a dynamic and changing process. The early phase is one of inflammation, followed by formation of granulation tissue and subsequent tissue remodelling and scarring. Simple cutaneous incisional wounds heal by first intention. Large cutaneous wounds heal by second intention, generating a significant amount of scar tissue. Healing is modified by a number of known influences and some unknown ones, influencing the quality and adequacy of both inflammation and repair. These influences include both *systemic* and *local host factors*. Local factors that influence healing include the following:

- *Infection* is the single most important cause of delay in healing because it results in persistent tissue injury and inflammation.
- *Mechanical factors*, can delay healing, by compressing blood vessels and separating the edges of the wound.
- *Foreign bodies*, constitute impediments to healing.
- *Size, location and type of wound influence healing*: wounds in richly vascularised areas, such as the face, heal faster than those in poorly vascularised ones, such as the foot. Small incisional injuries heal faster and with less scar formation than large excisional wounds or wounds caused by blunt trauma.

Systemic factors include the following:
- *Nutrition* has profound effects on wound healing. Protein deficiency, and particularly vitamin C deficiency, inhibit collagen synthesis and retard healing.
- *Metabolic status* can affect wound healing. Diabetes mellitus, is associated with delayed healing, as a consequence of the microangiopathy that is a frequent feature of this disease.
- *Circulatory status* can influence wound healing. *An inadequate blood supply*, usually caused by arteriosclerosis or venous abnormalities (e.g. varicose veins) that retard venous drainage, also impairs healing.
- *Hormones,* such as *glucocorticoids*, have anti-inflammatory effects that influence various components of inflammation. These agents also inhibit collagen synthesis.

CHAPTER 1 – ANSWERS

Trauma and Burns

Answer 1

(a) Glasgow Coma Scale (see Comment) *(2 marks)*

(b) BP, pulse and respiration
Pupillary sizes and reflexes
Eye movements (extrinsic muscles)
Abdominal reflexes; cremasteric reflex
Limbs:
   Tone, clonus
   Power
   Reflexes (triceps, biceps, brachioradialis, knee jerk,
   ankle jerk, plantar reflex) *(3 marks)*

(c) (i) Extra(epi)dural
    Subdural
    Subarachnoid
    Intracerebral
    CT/MRI of the head *(2 marks)*
  (ii) Protect airway and ventilate as necessary
    Exclude injury to cervical spine
    Record BP and pulse, with head injury
    observations quarter-hourly
    Daily ABGs
    FBC and U&Es
    Intracranial pressure (ICP) monitoring
    Mannitol infusion preoperatively
    Surgical evacuation of haematoma with
    placement of ICP monitoring device
    Postoperative antibiotic therapy *(3 marks)*

Comment

Glasgow Coma Scale		Score
Eyes open	Spontaneous	4/5
	To speech	3/4
	To pain	2
	None	1
Verbal response	Orientated	5
	Confused	4
	Inappropriate	3
	Incomprehensible	2
	None	1
Motor response	Obeys commands	5
	Localises pain	4
	Flexion to pain	3
	Extension to pain	2
	None	1
Best total score		14/15

In all forms of intracranial bleeding, the time between injury and decompression is a major determinant of outcome. The onus should, therefore, be on rapid evacuation to a neurosurgical centre for appropriate management.

Recovery from surgical evacuation of intracranial haematoma is slow and unpredictable. The multidisciplinary rehabilitation team should include neurosurgical, psychiatric, speech and language therapy and physiotherapy, and social and community services.

Answer 2

(a) Clinically assess airway patency and air exchange, namely the oropharynx, for foreign body or mucus plug obstruction, and respiratory movements. Monitor pulse and BP. Establish peripheral and central venous access for CVP, ABGs and pulmonary arterial wedge pressure measurements; FBC and U&Es. Administer O_2 by facemask. Record ECG *(3 marks)*

(b) Tension/open pneumothorax (including flail chest)
Massive haemothorax
Cardiac tamponade   *(2 marks)*

(c) (i)   Promptly close defect in chest wall with sterile
occlusive dressings large enough to overlap
wound edges and tape securely on three sides to
provide a flutter valve effect. Site a chest drain
remote from the wound. Close the wound
surgically when the patient's condition is
stable   *(2 marks)*

(ii) Decide drain site on chest radiograph, usually at
the fifth intercostal space from the midaxillary
line. Infiltrate area with lidocaine (1 or 2%) or
bupivacaine (0.5%). Make skin incision, enter
pleural cavity by blunt dissection, and introduce
tube drain on introducer into pleural cavity.
Connect drain to underwater
seal. Secure drain and close wound around
it with non-absorbable sutures   *(3 marks)*

Comment

Flail chest occurs when a segment of the chest wall becomes
detached from the ribcage. It leads to 'paradoxical breathing' but
may initially be masked as a result of splinting of the chest wall from
pain. Mechanical ventilation is usually indicated.

Massive haemothorax results from a rapid loss of 1–2 litres blood
into the pleural cavity and must be suspected when shock is
associated with absent breath sounds and dullness to percussion on
that side. Initial management is by simultaneous restoration of
blood volume and decompression of the pleural cavity. Continued
blood loss (>200 ml/h) may require thoracotomy.

Cardiac tamponade presents as paradoxical elevation of the jugular
venous pressure (JVP) on inspiration, fall in arterial pulse pressure
and muffled heart sounds (Beck's triad). Pericardiocentesis is
indicated when response to resuscitation is poor and the diagnosis
suspected. Tracings on a cardiac monitor may reveal injury patterns

that, along with a positive pericardiocentesis, would require thoracotomy and inspection of the heart.

Answer 3

(a) (i) Right-sided tension pneumothorax
Right haemothorax *(2 marks)*

(ii) Tracheal shift to left
Hyper-resonant or dull to percussion, with diminished or absent breath sounds in the right chest
Evidence of injury to chest wall on gently springing the ribcage *(2 marks)*

(b) (i) ABGs *(1 mark)*
(ii) Posteroanterior and lateral chest radiographs *(1 mark)*

(c) Pulmonary contusion
Myocardial contusion
Aortic disruption
Diaphragmatic rupture
Tracheobronchial disruption
Oesophageal disruption *(4 marks)*

Comment

Pulmonary and myocardial contusions are the most common potentially lethal chest injuries. In the former, respiratory failure may be subtle and develop over time and in the latter the diagnosis is made by abnormalities on the ECG. Traumatic aortic rupture is a cause of sudden death; potential survivors tend to have a laceration near the ligamentum anteriosum of the aorta, continuity being maintained by an intact adventitial layer. Many survivors die in hospital if the injury goes unrecognised. A cardinal radiological sign is a widened mediastinum, caused by the haematoma surrounding the aorta. Blunt traumatic disruption to the tracheobronchial tree, oesophagus and diaphragm may all present late, and operative repair with drainage is life saving.

Unlike immediately life-threatening conditions these injuries may not be obvious on initial examination, and timely diagnosis is often based on a high index of clinical suspicion.

Answer 4

(a) (i) Liver, spleen, pancreas, duodenum, diaphragm, kidneys, urinary bladder *(2 marks)*

    (ii) Ultrasonography or CT of abdomen *(1 mark)*

(b) (i) Quarter-hourly BP, pulse and respiration
Check urine for blood
Half-hourly urine output; catheterise if required
FBC, ABGs, chest and abdominal radiographs
(2 marks)

    (ii) Peripheral and central venous access for volume replacement and CVP monitoring. Intubation and mechanical ventilation for respiratory decompensation *(2 marks)*

(c) Developing signs of peritonism and an increase in abdominal girth signify intraperitoneal haemorrhage or rupture of a hollow viscus. Imaging of the abdomen or a diagnostic peritoneal lavage would detect bleeding and/or visceral injuries before the onset of lethal complications (oligaemia and/or toxic shock) *(3 marks)*

Comment

Unrecognised abdominal injury remains a frequent cause of preventable death after trauma. Peritoneal signs are often overshadowed by pain from associated injuries. Contrast-enhanced abdominal/pelvic CT scan is diagnostic. Diagnostic peritoneal lavage under local anaesthetic reveals the presence of intraperitoneal bleeding or bowel contents. A laparoscopic examination under a general anaesthetic may be useful when a significant visceral injury is suspected. It will confirm the diagnosis and determine the extent of the injury and the need for surgery.

Answer 5

(a) Resuscitation order:
Ensure airway patency and adequate ventilation by administering supplementary oxygen; intubate and ventilate manually if necessary
Immobilise cervical spine and place patient on a long spine board
Restore circulatory blood volume by crystalloids, plasma expanders and colloids as necessary, with pulse, BP and CVP monitoring
Commence head injury observations
Alleviate pain with opiate analgesics
Perform careful and thorough physical examination *(5 marks)*

(b) Counter hypothermia, administer O_2 and support ventilation, set up an intravenous infusion and maintain normal BP. Maintain constant verbal and tactile communication and reassure the conscious patient
Treat life- and limb-threatening emergencies as facilities permit (e.g. close open chest wound with occlusive dressing, control external haemorrhage with pressure dressing, realign displaced limb fractures) *(3 marks)*

(c) One anaesthetist
One trauma surgeon
One trauma nurse
One paramedic
One pilot
(Helicopter capacity rarely exceeds six people, including the patient and equipment) *(2 marks)*

Comment

Resuscitation is best carried out in the ambulance, except in respiratory or cardiac arrest, when intubation and external cardiac massage are performed at the roadside. When immediate extraction of the victim from the wreckage is not possible, life support is continued and consideration given to the need for on-site amputation of a severely injured trapped limb.

Answer 6

(a) Cervical spine: fracture of vertebral arches or bodies with/without dislocation
Cervical cord: concussion, incomplete lesion, hemisection, transection *(2 marks)*

(b) (i) Skin bruising on the lateral and/or posterior aspects of the neck; neck muscle spasm *(1 mark)*
(ii) Attempt to elicit passive movement! *(1 mark)*

(c) (i) Reduction and stabilisation of fracture by cervical traction or internal fixation in selected patients *(2 marks)*
(ii) Care of nutritional requirements and prevention of catabolic state
Prevention and treatment of respiratory and/or urinary infections
Skin care to prevent pressure sores
Physiotherapy to prevent joint contractures *(4 marks)*

Comment

Patients with suspected spinal injuries must be assessed after immobilisation on a long spine board with a semi-rigid collar and sand bag support to head, neck and shoulders. Cervical spine injuries are caused by flexion, rotation, compression and hyperextension. Indication for surgery is progression of neurological deficit despite reduction and external stabilisation. Spinal fusion avoids prolonged bedrest with its associated morbidity.

Answer 7

(a) (i) Use 'rule of nines' (modified for infants and toddlers)
Affected area: approximately 18%   *(1 mark)*

(ii) Verbal reassurance
Pain relief and sedation
Tetanus prophylaxis
Wound toilet: the burn surface is either left exposed or covered with dressing impregnated with silver nitrate or an antibiotic in an oil or water base
Prophylactic antibiotic therapy for 5–10 days   *(4 marks)*

(b) (i) Partial-thickness injury appears moist, red and blistered, with preservation of pain sensation

Full-thickness injury is usually white or brown, dry, firm and insensitive to touch   *(2 marks)*

(ii) The equation [Body weight (kg) × Percentage burned surface = Amount of fluid (ml)] gives the amount required in the first 4 hours. Monitor haematocrit and hourly urine output and give same amount over next 4 hours. Provided that the clinical state is stable, give the same amount over the next 16 hours. (Approximately half colloid and half crystalloid solutions)   *(3 marks)*

Comment

The child may develop paralytic ileus and for the first 6–8 hours the oral intake should be restricted to 50 ml water/hour, and thereafter gradually increased to half-strength milk, followed by a liquid diet.

Immediate tangential excision of the burn with split-skin grafting reduces fluid and protein loss, prevents infection and accelerates healing.

CHAPTER 2 – ANSWERS

Answer 8

(a) (i) Smoke inhalation injury (respiratory tract burns) *(1 mark)*

    (ii) Humidified oxygen by facemask
Ambu-Bag ventilation if required
Calm patient with reassurance
Mild sedation if necessary *(2 marks)*

(b) (i) Laryngeal oedema and/or oedema of the lower respiratory tract with bronchospasm *(2 marks)*

    (ii) Endotracheal intubation with assisted ventilation
Tracheostomy, if prolonged mechanical ventilation is required *(2 marks)*

    (iii) Relieve bronchospasm with bronchodilators and steroids (as required)
Positive pressure ventilation if ABGs deteriorate
Prophylactic systemic antibiotic cover
Intravenous crystalloid administration to maintain hydration and renal function *(3 marks)*

Comment

Failure of oral intubation requires emergency cricothyroidotomy and tracheal intubation because severe respiratory burns lead rapidly to respiratory failure and death. Lesser degrees of bronchial and alveolar damage lead to the 'shock lung syndrome', with increased airway resistance, raised pulmonary arterial wedge pressure and right ventricular strain. Cardiopulmonary support in an intensive therapy unit is needed until lung function recovers.

Answer 9

(a) (i) Apply semi-rigid cervical collar
Support spine during lifting and log-rolling
Strap patient in a neutral position on a long spine board for transfer to hospital, with sand bags to support head, neck and shoulders *(2 marks)*

(ii) A lateral radiograph showing the base of the skull, all seven cervical vertebrae and the first thoracic vertebra
An anteroposterior (AP) neck radiograph to include an open mouth odontoid view
An AP view of the dorsal spine *(2 marks)*

(b) Flaccid areflexia, especially with a flaccid rectal sphincter
Diaphragmatic breathing
Passive flexion but not extension at the elbow
Grimaces to painful stimuli above but not below the clavicle
Hypotension with bradycardia
Priapism (an uncommon but characteristic sign) *(3 marks)*

(c) Neurogenic shock results from injury to descending sympathetic pathways in the spinal cord, with loss of vasomotor tone and sympathetic innervation to the heart. The former causes intravascular pooling of blood and consequent hypotension, and the latter inability to increase the heart rate, producing bradycardia. The BP, therefore, cannot be restored by fluid infusion alone, and the judicious use of vasopressor agents may be required *(3 marks)*

Comment

Three tracts are readily assessed clinically in evaluating a spinal cord injury. The corticospinal tract controls motor power on the same side and is tested by voluntary muscle contractions or involuntary response to painful stimuli. The spinothalamic tract transmits pain and temperature sensations to the opposite side and is tested by pinch or pinprick. The posterior columns carry proprioceptive impulses from the same side and are tested by position sense of the fingers and toes or tuning fork vibrations. A complete spinal cord lesion abolishes distal neurological function and prognosis for recovery is poor. Incomplete spinal cord lesions are compatible with recovery, and a careful examination to determine the presence of any sensory or motor function is, therefore, essential.

Answer 10

(a) (i) Primary survey detects tracheal deviation and rib injury (by gently springing the ribcage) and the presence of:
Central cyanosis
Paradoxical breathing
Surgical emphysema
Abdominal skin bruising or tenderness
Chest radiograph   *(2 marks)*

(ii) Plain AP view of the pelvis, ultrasonography and/or CT of abdomen and pelvis and/or diagnostic peritoneal lavage or laparoscopic examination
Catheterise and examine urine for blood   *(2 marks)*

(iii) Gentle palpation for a fracture and/or dislocation
AP and lateral radiographs of the hip, femur, knee, tibia, fibula and ankle   *(2 marks)*

(b) Establish two large-calibre intravenous peripheral lines
Establish a central venous line for CVP monitoring
Send blood for FBC, ABGs, grouping and emergency crossmatch
Transfuse with crystalloid solution (e.g. Ringer's lactate) and a plasma volume expander (e.g. Haemaccel) until whole blood is available to restore blood volume   *(4 marks)*

Comment

The pulse and BP are monitored quarter-hourly, although these are poor measures of tissue perfusion. A pulse oximeter measures the saturation of haemoglobin colorimetrically (it is not a measure of P_{O_2}); a small sensor is clipped on to the finger, toe or earlobe, and displays the pulse rate and oxygen concentration continuously in addition to reflecting the respiratory and circulatory status.

Hypovolaemic shock may not respond to fluid therapy alone. Once the circulatory blood volume has been replaced, and if tissue perfusion has not recovered as a result of peripheral vascular shutdown, judicious use of steroids and pressor agents to maintain renal and cerebral perfusion may be appropriate in an intensive care setting.

Answer 11

(a) Extent: chest and abdomen make up 18% and each arm 7% of total body surface area ('rule of nines' modified for infants and toddlers)
Depth: partial-thickness (epidermal) scald blanches on pressure, is pink and may blister, and is painful to pinprick
Full-thickness scald does not blanch, is pale or dull brown, and is devoid of pain (negative pinprick)   *(3 marks)*

(b) Scalds exceeding 10% of body surface or a full-thickness scald exceeding 2.5 cm^2
Unrelated but significant underlying illness, e.g. diabetes, heart disease or epilepsy
Injury suspected of being non-accidental
Poor home circumstances   *(3 marks)*

(c) Open method: expose surface moistened with antibacterial agents, in an environment of sterile ambient air
Closed method: cover area with sterile, occlusive, non-adherent dressings impregnated with antibacterial agents, which are: chlorhexidine-impregnated tulle gras, which has anti-staphylococcal action; 1% sulfadiazine cream, which has anti-Gram-negative action (e.g. *Pseudomonas* and *Klebsiella* spp., *Escherichia coli*); 10% sulphamylon cream, which has same spectrum as above but penetrates avascular tissue; 0.5% silver nitrate solution soaked in cotton gauze, which is bacteriostatic   *(4 marks)*

Comment
Details of the circumstances of the injury must be obtained from
an accompanying adult. The temperature of the liquid, whether
clothing was worn, the exposure time, and whether the surface was
cooled with tap water or cold milk soon afterwards are important
in assessing wound depth and prognosis. The time interval
between scalding and presentation, if more than 6 hours, is likely
to result in an infection. Tetanus prophylaxis or immunisation is
administered on presentation; pain relief, sedation and oral intake
after intravenous hydration is monitored in the ensuing days.
Bacterial colonisation of the injured surface is usually complete in
24–48 h. This colonisation may manifest as a local infection or
result in systemic spread, with fever and rigors. Prophylactic
antibiotic therapy is therefore indicated in scalds exceeding 10% of
the surface.

Answer 12

(a) Airway patency and respiratory function (A + B)
      Cardiac function by recording the pulse, BP and
      electrical activity on a cardiac monitor (C)
      Level of consciousness: GCS score chart (D)   *(3 marks)*

(b) Full-thickness burn wounds at entry and exit sites with
      variable underlying tissue destruction and damage to
      intervening tissue, namely subcutaneous fat and
      muscle   *(3 marks)*

(c) Heart: ectopic rhythms, arrhythmias, ventricular
      fibrillation leading to cardiac arrest
      Kidneys: acute renal failure as a result of: (1) reduced
      perfusion during the shock phase; or (2) released Hb
      from red cells and damaged muscle
      Muscle: tetanic contractions leading to joint and soft
      tissue injuries
      Brain: convulsions leading to cerebral oedema
      Peripheral nerves: conduction defects   *(4 marks)*

Comment

The ABCDE of primary assessment is followed. Immediate cardiopulmonary resuscitation is commenced in ventricular arrhythmias. ECG monitoring and cardiac enzyme estimations detect injury to the heart muscle. Tissue destruction in high-voltage electrical injuries is extensive and may progress as initially viable tissue necroses, resulting from vascular thrombosis and capillary damage. In addition to wound débridement, excision of dead or poorly viable muscle is required to prevent myoglobinuria and gas gangrene. Wounds must be left open, because progressive muscle necrosis is likely and may require further débridement. Early fasciotomy may be required if limb swelling progresses, to preserve its blood supply. Sustained diuresis is required to prevent renal failure from the breakdown products of muscle damage.

Answer 13

(a) The loss of serous fluid from the burned surface is replaced by plasma in the form of plasma protein fraction (PPF) or fresh-frozen plasma (FFP) in 4-hourly aliquots calculated as follows:

Percentage burn area × Patient's body weight × ½ (ml)

This initial guide is modified by the clinical, haematological and biochemical profiles during the 24-hour period *(3 marks)*

(b) Wound débridement and toilet

Keep wound surface warm and moist with open or closed methods

Take wound culture swabs from multiple sites daily

Cover burned area early by homografts or heterografts that are renewed in the ward until the entire area has received autografts from the patient's own donor sites

Correct dehydration, hypoproteinaemia and anaemia

Ensure adequate oral nutritional intake *(4 marks)*

CHAPTER 2 – ANSWERS

(c)   Ensure adequate pain relief with intravenous opiates
and optimal fluid and electrolyte balance

The patient may only have a few hours of clarity of
thought left before lapsing into confusion or coma.
Therefore, explain the probable outcome and prognosis
and the therapeutic options gently and dispassionately
so that the patient's wishes on further management
may be adhered to. Maximise time spent with loved
ones and relatives with ready access to a counsellor or
priest. Seclude the patient from extraneous ward
activity.   *(3 marks)*

Comment

The extent of the burn injury is estimated using the 'rule of nines'.
The depth of the burn should be mapped out and may be broadly
divided into superficial (partial thickness) or deep (full
thickness). The former involves the epidermis and superficial
layers of the dermis and, in the latter, the epidermis and dermis
are destroyed with a variable extent of underlying tissue. A third
type that is occasionally seen is the deep dermal burn, where some
of the germinal layers are spared but healing is poor and
protracted, with wound contracture and scarring. Flame burns
are almost always deep, and the burn surface is débrided by
tangential excision and covered by 'split-skin' grafts taken from
the patient's own donor sites.

However, when the burn area is larger than the available donor
sites, banked cadaver or pig skin may be used as temporary
dressings until the area is grafted in stages using the patient's own
skin. The former must be renewed every few days to prevent
adherence and bleeding. There is no reliable evidence that using
such 'other skin' dressings is superior to conventional antiseptic-
impregnated, non-adherent gauze. Survival after a burn injury
depends on the patient's age, and the burn area and depth. In very
young, very old and chronically ill individuals, the morbidity is
high, from complications of the burn injury.

Answer 14

(a) Patient 2, patient 1, patient 4, patient 3, patient 5

(3 marks)

(b) Patient 2: severe head injury; in acute respiratory distress as a result of airway compromise; requires urgent airway control (A) and ventilatory support (B), volume replacement (C) and neurological assessment (D)

Patient 1: probable crush injury to the chest with major limb fractures; requires A and B and C

Patient 4: probable cervical spine injury with cord compression/damage; requires urgent stabilisation on a spine board (A) and neurological assessment (D)

Patient 3: uterine trauma with probable fetal distress; requires fetal monitoring and sedation

Patient 5: bilateral ankle fractures and probable fracture/dislocation of the right hip *(7 marks)*

Comment

In the severely injured patient the 'golden hour' after injury is when resuscitatory measures have far-reaching effects on outcome and morbidity. Severe injuries kill or maim in specific reproducible timeframes. Thus ABCD or resuscitation prioritises the assessment and resuscitation of organ systems in the following order:

- A Airway with cervical spine control
- B Breathing
- C Circulation
- D Disability (neurological).

Answer 15

(a) Patient 2, patient 4, patient 3, patient 5, patient 1
(3 marks)

(b) Patient 2: external haemorrhage; internal injuries/bleeding; requires urgent volume replacement (C), cervical spine control (A) and head injury assessment (D)

Patient 4: flail segment right ribcage with probable tension pneumothorax and lung collapse; probable crush injury to the abdomen; requires urgent A and B and C

Patient 3: crush injuries and fractures of both lower limbs; will be hypovolaemic; requires pain relief, volume replacement and assessment of lower limb perfusion (C); renal function requires close monitoring

Patient 5: severe psychological trauma; appears not be have suffered physical injury; requires full injury survey and sedation

Patient 1: asphyxiated (A, B) with cerebral anoxia (D) and hypovolaemia (C) with cardiac failure; unlikely to respond to resuscitation　　*(7 marks)*

Comment

Active resuscitation of patients with a low priority alongside those of a higher priority depends on the clinical resources available. However, in patients with a poor expectation of survival, active measures may be abandoned only after a negative or unsustainable physiological response to resuscitation. The time lapse between the injury and the start of resuscitation largely determines the outcome of severe injuries. This is particularly true of victims of natural disasters when long delays may be inevitable, where communication and transport systems are disrupted, and rescue efforts require the mobilisation of rescue teams with logistic support.

Answer 16

(a) Patient 5, patient 2, patient 4, patient 1, patient 3

(3 marks)

(b) Patient 5, despite the absence of external burns, has smoke inhalation with compromised alveolar gaseous exchange resulting in cerebral hypoxia; requires urgent airway control (A) and assisted ventilation with oxygen therapy (B) to improve cerebral oxygenation (D) and for the management of the 'shock lung syndrome'

Patient 2: fracture of the shoulder girdle with a suspected cervical spine injury; requires urgent spinal immobilisation (A) and pain relief

Patient 4: is hypovolaemic from blood loss and requires control of bleeding from lacerations (volume replacement and analgesic)

Patient 1: significant surface burn area, inhalation injury and blood loss from the scalp laceration; requires urgent ventilatory support and oxygen therapy (B), volume replacement (C) and pain control *(7 marks)*

Patient 3: 65% surface burns and inhalation injury with cerebral hypoxia at the age of 72 suggests a poor prognostic outcome despite intensive therapy

Comment

Clinical evidence of an inhalation injury from heat or fumes can be a history of explosion or confinement in a burning environment, facial burns, singeing of eyebrows or nasal vibrissae, hoarseness or coughing up of carbonaceous sputum, acutely inflamed oropharynx and impaired cerebration. Carbon monoxide poisoning must be assumed in these patients and assisted ventilation and oxygen therapy instituted urgently.

Answer 17

(a)   All medical teams on call
      All laboratory personnel on call
      Head of nursing and patient services
      Chief pharmacist
      Medical director
      Chief administrator (chief executive officer)
      Switchboard operator on duty would summon the
      above when instructed to put the disaster plan
      into action (includes key clinical staff not on call)
                                                        (3 marks)

(b)   Emergency Department foyer as the reception area for
      all casualties
      Emergency Department as the red-coded area
      Day surgery unit as the yellow-coded area
      Outpatient department as the blue-coded area
      Hospital foyer as the reception area for relatives
      and the media   *(3 marks)*

(c)   Casualties are received and triaged into three colour-
      coded categories, as follows:
      •   Red: critically injured and those with severe injuries
          requiring urgent resuscitation
      •   Yellow: moderately severe, non-life-threatening
          injuries
      •   Blue: minor injuries, i.e. the 'walking wounded'
          and those with post-traumatic stress symptoms
                                                        (4 marks)

Comment

A major incident calls for the immediate implementation of the
emergency disaster plan. This involves the immediate mobilisation
of predetermined hospital personnel (including those not on duty
at the time) to the designated reception and treatment areas; a
senior clinician is nominated to coordinate operations in each
area. The group allocated to the reception area assesses and triages
patients to the treatment areas coded red, yellow and blue. The
transfer of patients requiring specialised care to regional centres

after stabilisation is coordinated by a senior clinician. Beds are to be made available for those requiring admission and may involve the transfer of convalescent inpatients to other hospitals. A senior manager arranges technical and catering services to be made available to patients and staff.

Answer 18

(a) Pelvic fracture with urethral injury   *(2 marks)*

(b) The clinical signs in pelvic fracture include:
- Tenderness over the pelvis that can be appreciated with pelvic springing indicates fracture. Pelvic springing involves applying alternating gentle compression and distortion over the iliac wings
- Palpable instability of the pelvis on bimanual compression or distraction of the iliac wings also indicates fracture. Be very gentle when pelvic tenderness is appreciated. Do not rock or apply great force until radiographs exclude skeletally unstable pelvic fractures, because an overly aggressive examination can increase haemorrhage unnecessarily. Likewise, examination should be limited to one examiner. Remember that, in the later stages of pregnancy, the pelvic ligaments become stretched and may mimic instability
- Instability on hip adduction and pain on hip motion suggest an acetabular fracture (in addition to possible hip fracture)
- Signs of urethral injury in males include a high-riding or boggy prostate on rectal examination, scrotal haematoma or blood at the urethral meatus
- Vaginal bleeding or palpable fracture line on careful bimanual examination suggests pelvic fracture in females
- Other signs of pelvic fracture include the following:
  - haematuria
  - rectal bleeding or Earle's sign, the appreciation of a large haematoma or palpable fracture line on careful rectal examination

Destot's sign: a haematoma above the inguinal
ligament, on the proximal thigh or over the perineum

Grey Turner's sign: a flank ecchymosis associated with
retroperitoneal bleeding:

- Roux sign: a bilateral asymmetry in the
  distances between the greater trochanter and the
  pubic spine on each side (indicating an
  overriding fracture of the anterior pelvic ring)
- neurovascular deficits of the lower
  extremities   *(4 marks)*

(c) Immediate complications include pelvic haemorrhage,
     bladder injury, urethral injury, and nerve injury
     involving sacral plexus, sacral nerve roots or
     sciatic nerve   *(2 marks)*

(d) Although pelvic radiograph is mandatory (ATLS
     guideline) in trauma patients with suspected organ
     injuries a contrast enhanced CT of the pelvis and
     abdomen is needed to assess subtle fractures and
     disruptions. In particular, sacral fractures can be
     difficult to detect on radiographs.   *(2 marks)*

Comments

Pelvic fracture is a disruption of the bony structure of the pelvis.
The most common cause in elderly people is a fall, but the most
significant fractures involve high-energy forces such as a motor
vehicle accident or a fall from significant height. Diagnosis is made
on the basis of history, clinical features and special investigations,
usually including radiographs and CT.

The complication rate is significant and related to injury of the
underlying organs and bleeding. As a result of the tremendous
force necessary to cause most unstable pelvic fractures,
concomitant severe injuries are common and are associated with
high morbidity and mortality rates. In addition, pelvic fractures
increase the incidence of pulmonary emboli. The overall mortality
rate is about 10% in adults and 5% in children. Pelvic
haemorrhage is the direct cause of death in fewer than half the

patients with pelvic fractures who die. Retroperitoneal haemorrhage and secondary infection are the main causes of death in children and adults with pelvic fractures. If hypotension is present on arrival to the Emergency Department, the mortality rate approaches 50%. If the fracture is open, the mortality rate reaches 30%.

Emergency treatment consists of ATLS management. After stabilisation, the pelvis may be surgically reconstructed.

3

Orthopaedics

Answer 1

(a) Plain radiology of the femur and knee joint
Open biopsy of the lesion *(2 marks)*

(b) Ewing's sarcoma
Chondroblastoma
Osteosarcoma *(3 marks)*

(c) Counselling the child and parents/carers with regard to treatment, reconstructive surgery or prosthetic fitting
Preoperative radiotherapy
Radical surgery with complete tumour resection
Limb reconstruction or prosthetic fitting
Adjuvant chemotherapy *(5 marks)*

Comment

Osteosarcoma and chondroblastoma rarely present with constitutional symptoms, whereas Ewing's sarcoma, which arises in the diaphysis or metaphysis of the long bones, may give rise to malaise, pyrexia and a raised ESR, simulating osteomyelitis. Radiological appearances of these tumours show new bone formation with 'sun-ray' spicules of new bone or subperiosteal new bone formation, alongside areas of bone destruction. Radiotherapy and/or chemotherapy may precede surgery to control metastatic spread and produce tumour regression. Radical surgery, the mainstay of treatment, may be accompanied by reconstruction of the bone and the adjacent joint with prosthetic implants or bone allografts to restore function and appearance.

Answer 2

(a) Lumbar intervertebral disc prolapse/protrusion, traumatic or degenerative in origin; rupture of the fibrous covering of the disc leads to herniation of the disc pulp into the spinal canal, causing compression of the nerve roots that issue from the intervertebral foramina above and below the prolapsed disc; spinal canal tumours and metastatic tumour deposits are rare causes of nerve root irritation   (*3 marks*)

(b) Pain and/or sensory loss in:
- the groin suggests first lumbar root
- the front of the mid or lower thigh with quadriceps muscle weakness and diminished knee jerk suggests second and third lumbar roots
- the back or side of the thigh, lateral aspect of the leg and dorsum of the foot, with quadriceps and anterior tibial muscle weakness and diminished knee jerk, suggest fourth and fifth lumbar roots

In addition, sensory loss:
- over the dorsum of the foot and specific weakness on dorsiflexion of the great toe suggest fifth root
- in the sole of the foot, weakness on plantar flexion and an absent ankle jerk suggest first sacral root compression   (*3 marks*)

(c) Initial measures are complete bedrest, analgesia and muscle relaxants; if symptoms do not settle or there is neurological deterioration or involvement of sphincter function, spinal CT or MRI may delineate the site of cord/root compression requiring surgical decompression. This may involve microdisectomy or an open laminectomy, removing the debris in the intervertebral disc space and freeing the nerve roots. Spinal fusion may be required to stabilise the spine
            (*4 marks*)

CHAPTER 3 – ANSWERS

Comment

The clinical picture of lumbar disc prolapse is initial back pain, which later radiates to the leg; with nerve root compression there is skin paraesthesia, muscle cramps and tenderness, progressing to sensory loss and motor weakness. If urinary and/or anal sphincter tone is compromised ('cauda equina' syndrome), emergency surgical decompression is required.

Answer 3

  (a) Loosening of the prosthesis
       Dislocation of the prosthesis
       Osteomyelitis of the surgical site   *(3 marks)*

  (b) Clinical examination:
       Overlying tissue induration and joint tenderness
       Sinus formation
       Limb shortening
       Restriction of movements
      Plain radiology of the joint:
       Prosthetic dislocation
       Prosthetic loosening
       Prosthetic migration
       Bone resorption osteomyelitis   *(3 marks)*

  (c) Poor surgical technique: bone infection, misplacement, nerve and muscle damage
       Flawed prosthetic material: loosening or fracture of prosthesis, rapid wear of components as a result of foreign body reaction
       Bone demineralisation: fracture at site of implant
                                        (4 marks)

Comment

Hip replacement surgery is now commonplace, with long patient waiting lists for the procedure; complications of surgery are becoming increasingly familiar to carers outside as well as within the orthopaedic speciality. Joint replacement is designed to relieve pain and provide a degree of mobility with a functional lifespan of

15–20 years; the complications become increasingly prevalent with the passage of time. The development of precision implants that do not require cement may improve long-term results.

Answer 4

(a) (i) Hallux valgus deformity with inflammatory arthritis of the first metatarsophalangeal joint *(2 marks)*

(ii) Symptoms are caused by pressure/friction on the medial aspect of the first metatarsal head, producing joint deviation, exostosis formation and arthritis *(2 marks)*

(b) Habitual wearing of narrow, unyielding, raised heel shoes that produce progressive lateral deviation of the big toe *(2 marks)*

(c) Surgery for hallux valgus is designed to correct the deformity and preserve the function of the big toe; this is achieved by excision of the medial bony prominence, division of the contracted abductor muscle of the first web space, tightening of the stretched medial collateral ligament and realignment of the first metatarsal shaft by wedge osteotomy *(4 marks)*

Comment

Conservative measures to correct hallux valgus deformity by changing to shoes with wide fronts and low heels are generally unsatisfactory, because of poor patient compliance. In severe deformities there is over- or under-riding of the second toe by the first. The former may produce a painful dorsal callosity on the second toe, or it may be displaced to impinge with and cross the third toe.

Answer 5

(a) Cervical spondylosis: this is a degenerative disease producing osteophytes that project into the intervertebral foramen; sudden neck movements or strain may precipitate symptoms, produced by the narrowed foramen on the issuing nerve root   *(3 marks)*

(b) The lesion usually affects the nerve roots at C5–6 or C6–7 intervertebral joints to produce the following clinical picture: pain and/or sensory loss over shoulder tip, upper arm and dorsum of forearm (fingers are affected in C7 root involvement); weakness of trapezius, biceps and forearm extensors; and diminished biceps, triceps and supinator reflexes   *(3 marks)*

(c) Mild symptoms may be controlled by a semi-rigid collar, analgesics and muscle relaxants; progressive neurological signs may require an anterior decompression (disectomy) or laminectomy, with stabilisation of the cervical spine with bone grafts or prosthetic implant to preserve disk space   *(4 marks)*

Comment

Cervical spondylosis may be asymptomatic and come to light only after neck trauma. Measures to relieve muscle spasm by partially immobilising the cervical spine are usually sufficient until the inflammation produced by the injury subsides. Progressive root compression affecting the use of that limb is an indication for surgical decompression.

Answer 6

(a) Muscle spasm resulting in restricted range of movements, namely of abduction and internal rotation. A soft tissue swelling may be present   *(3 marks)*

(b) (i) Perthes' disease, slipped upper femoral epiphysis and tuberculosis (TB) of the hip *(2 marks)*

(ii) Perthes' disease (osteochondritis of the femoral epiphysis): collapse/fragmentation of ossification centre resulting in flattening of femoral head

Slipped upper femoral epiphysis: displacement of femoral epiphysis

TB of the hip: loss of bone density adjacent to joint with narrowing of joint space; later, bone destruction, with abscess formation *(2 marks)*

(c) In Perthes' disease and slipped epiphysis, avascular necrosis leads to progressive deformity and osteoarthritis in early adult life

In TB, complete destruction of the joint, with abscess and later sinus formation; systemic spread may lead to a fatal outcome *(3 marks)*

Comment

The pathogenesis of Perthes' disease and slipped upper femoral epiphysis is ischaemia of the femoral head. Both occur between age 5 and age 15 years, when the femoral head depends on the lateral epiphyseal vessels for its blood supply. TB of the hip joint is usually secondary to primary disease in the lung or bowel, and is accompanied by constitutional symptoms. A chest radiograph and positive Mantoux test are required to support the diagnosis.

Answer 7

(a) Injury depends on the extent of rotation and is progressive as follows: tear of anterior part of lateral ligament leads to fractures of the lateral malleolus and then the medial malleolus (bimalleolar fracture). Tear of the medial ligament leads to fracture of the posterior articular surface of the tibia, which may extend to a trimalleolar fracture dislocation (Pott's fracture) *(4 marks)*

CHAPTER 3 – ANSWERS

(b) Proximal fibular fracture with diastasis of the inferior tibiofibular joint and disruption of the interosseous tibiofibular ligament *(2 marks)*

(c) Principle: restoration of normal ankle mortice
Unstable ankle fractures may be treated with:
- external reduction and immobilisation in above-knee plaster cast; weight bearing is avoided for 4–6 weeks
- internal fixation: (this prevents late displacement) and early mobilisation *(4 marks)*

Comment

One of the most common diagnostic errors in ankle injuries is to miss a proximal fibular fracture; radiographs must include the knee and ankle joints. Failure of effective treatment of an ankle diastasis leads to permanent ankle instability.

Answer 8

(a) (i) Rheumatoid arthritis *(1 mark)*
(ii) Stage 1: synovitis – thickening of capsule, villous formation of synovium and a cell rich effusion into the joint and tendon sheaths
Stage 2: destruction – articular cartilage and tendon sheaths are eroded
Stage 3: deformity – the combination of articular destruction, capsular stretching and tendon rupture leads to progressive instability and deformity of the joint *(3 marks)*

(b) Normocytic/hypochromic anaemia
Rise in ESR, CRP and oncoproteins
Rheumatoid factor present in 80% and antinuclear factor in 30% of patients *(3 marks)*

(c) Stop synovitis, prevent deformity, reconstruct the joint and rehabilitate the patient, using a multidisciplinary approach *(3 marks)*

Comment

There is no cure for rheumatoid arthritis. Joint pain and swelling caused by the synovitis are reduced by bedrest and non-steroidal anti-inflammatory drugs (NSAIDs). Systemic corticosteroids give effective relief of symptoms but have serious side effects. Intrasynovial injections of corticosteroids and cytotoxic drugs reduce joint inflammation, as do systemically administered gold, penicillamine, hydroxychloroquine and methotrexate (immunosuppression). Joint splinting, physiotherapy and postural training may prevent progressive deformity. Deformity associated with loss of function and pain is treated by joint reconstruction or joint replacement. Bromolin found in pineapple is said to have anti-rheumatoid properties and regular consumption of the latter may ameliorate symptoms.

Answer 9

(a) Decreased joint space as a result of thinning of the cartilage
Subarticular sclerosis
Subchondral cyst formation
Osteophyte formation   *(3 marks)*

(b) Analgesics and warmth
NSAIDs
Preservation of movement by non-weight-bearing exercises
Adjustment of activities to reduce stress on the hip
                                   (3 marks)

(c) (i)   Progressive increase in pain
Severe restriction of activities
Marked deformity
Progressive loss of movement, in particular abduction
Radiological signs of joint destruction   *(3 marks)*
(ii) Total hip replacement   *(1 mark)*

Comment

Primary osteoarthritis is common in the fifth and sixth decades of life with an increased incidence in Caucasians. The articular cartilage becomes soft and fibrillated, and the underlying bone shows cyst formation and sclerosis. Synovial hypertrophy and capsular fibrosis cause joint stiffness. Realignment osteotomy may arrest or slow further cartilage destruction, whereas arthrodesis of the hip produces freedom from pain and stability, at the expense of mobility. Total replacement arthroplasty, replacing the acetabulum as well as the head of the femur, is the operation of choice.

Answer 10

(a) Closed reduction under general anaesthetic with longitudinal traction on the forearm, gradually flexing the elbow
Correct lateral displacement during traction
Monitor radial pulse throughout
Apply a back slab to flexed elbow, and a collar and cuff
Admit overnight to monitor limb circulation
Immobilise for 3 weeks   *(4 marks)*

(b) Ischaemia of forearm and hand as a result of arterial injury, arterial spasm or swelling of flexor compartment
Treatment: remove all dressings
Reduce fracture immediately
Do not overflex a badly swollen arm
If the radial pulse does not return, surgical decompression of the forearm and/or exploration of the brachial artery at the vicinity of the fracture
(3 marks)

(c) Injury to brachial artery/vein
Injury to nerves
Epiphyseal damage
Stiffness and delayed functional recovery
Volkmann's ischaemic contracture   *(3 marks)*

Comment

The importance of this fracture is the associated neurovascular injury. Monitoring the radial pulse during and immediately after reduction is of cardinal importance in avoiding ischaemic injury.

Pulse, hand sensation and finger movements must be monitored, overnight, to detect possible nerve or vessel compression. If closed reduction is not possible without compromising the brachial artery, open reduction or Dunlop traction (longitudinal traction via a pin in the olecranon) may be used.

Answer 11

(a) Colles' fracture   *(1 mark)*

(b) Scaphoid fracture, wrist dislocation, injuries to the elbow, humerus and shoulder, and an acute carpal tunnel syndrome may be associated with this fracture   *(3 marks)*

(c) The mainstay of investigation and diagnosis of the distal radial fracture is anteroposterior (AP) and lateral radiographs. These are used to make the diagnosis and classify the fracture. Deformity is assessed on both views by measurement of the dorsal angle, radial shift and degree of shortening of the distal radius. The fracture usually occurs about an inch or two (2.5–5 cm) proximal to the radiocarpal joint with posterior and lateral displacement of the distal fragment, resulting in the characteristic dinner fork-like deformity. Often the ulnar styloid process is also fractured   *(3 marks)*

(d) Malunion, nerve injury (commonly median nerve) and reflex sympathetic dystrophy are common complications associated with Colles' fracture   *(3 marks)*

Comment

A Colles' fracture is a fracture affecting the distal end of the radius and often the ulnar styloid. As a result of its close proximity to the wrist joint this injury is often called a wrist fracture. This is the most commonly occurring fracture in adults and is a common fragility fracture in elderly people, as well as being a common injury in children where it may involve the growth plate.

Investigation of a potential distal radial fracture includes assessment of the *lateral articular angle, radial length* and *articular surface* on plain AP and lateral radiographs.

The lateral articular angle is the angle between the axis of the radius and the articular cup. This angle is measured on radiographs. Normally, the angle is turned down towards the thumb (volar angulation) by 11°. As pressure is applied to the radius, the cup may become aligned differently. Alignment up to 0° is still considered to be functional, and does not require any intervention. However, angulation away from the thumb (dorsal angulation) beyond this point (> 11° deviation) requires reduction of the fracture. When dorsal angulation beyond the acceptable threshold occurs, distal radioulnar joint motion is altered and forearm rotation becomes restricted. The upper limit of an acceptable deformity after reduction of the fracture is 5° of dorsal angulation.

Radial length is one of the important considerations in a distal radius fracture. The core question that must be answered is 'is it short?' The radius length would be too short if there were more than neutral variance, especially when compared with the opposite side of the body. If the radial length remains uncorrected, ulnar impaction syndrome may occur.

Any articular joint surface must be smooth for it to function properly. The surface is not smooth if there is more than a 1–mm step deformity, and it is associated with post-traumatic arthrosis. Irregularity may result in radiocarpal arthritis, pain and stiffness. If the surface is very irregular, the optimal treatment is fusion.

Many factors have an influence on the choice of treatment for a distal radial fracture, including fracture characteristics such as amount of displacement, comminution, involvement of joints, bone quality and inherent instability. The patient's characteristics are also important: their age, level of activity, general health and functional needs, with the last three being more important than chronological age.

The initial treatment of a distal radial fracture depends on the degree of displacement. If the fracture is undisplaced or minimally displaced, it is sufficient to place the forearm in a cast with the wrist in the neutral position. The metacarpophalangeal joints and the thumb must be left free to mobilise.

In displaced fractures the requirement for reduction must be assessed. Functional deficit is likely to ensue if there is more than 10° of dorsal angulation or more than 15° of volar tilt or carpal malalignment, and these would seem to be reasonable indications for reduction.

Reduction is usually performed under regional anaesthesia or a local anaesthetic haematoma block. Regional anaesthesia is preferred because it allows better pain relief and improved reduction but it does have the disadvantage of requiring a second doctor in attendance.

Closed reduction using longitudinal manual traction is successful in about 95% of cases. Localised thumb pressure over the distal fragment with slight wrist flexion for dorsally displaced fractures, or extension for volar displaced fractures, can also be helpful.

Unstable fractures require external or internal fixation.

CHAPTER 3 – ANSWERS

Answer 12

   (a)   Ingrown toenail   *(1 mark)*

   (b)   The nailplate can be forced out of the nail groove by footwear with a toe box that is too small for the forefoot, by trauma or by cutting the nail back in a curvilinear fashion   *(3 marks)*

   (c)   Ingrown nails result from an alteration in the proper fit of the nailplate in the usual nail groove. Sharp spicules of the lateral nail margin develop and are gradually driven into the dermis of the nail groove. The nail acts as a foreign body. An inflammatory response occurs in the area of penetration, leading to erythema, oedema, purulence, and development of granulation tissue Development of ingrown nails is divided into three stages: (1) erythema, oedema and focal tenderness; (2) crusting and expressible purulence at the nailfold and nailplate junction; and (3) chronic infection with protuberant granulation tissue extending over the nailplate   *(2 marks)*

   (d)   Radiology may be appropriate to rule out fracture, foreign body or suspected osteomyelitis as indicated by history and physical examination   *(2 marks)*

   (e)   Treatment options depend on the stage of ingrown toenail:

         Stage 1 can be managed by recommending shoes with a comfortable wide toe box or open-toed shoes. Instruct the patient (or patient's parents if a child) to cut the nail straight across and avoid cutting back the lateral margins. The nail edge should extend past the tissue

         Stage 2 can be treated by stretching the soft tissue away from the side of the nail, elevating the offending edge of nail from the soft tissue, and placing a small pledget of cotton under the nail edge to lift it back into the nail grove. Instruct patients with stage 2 ingrown nails on how to perform this treatment. Parents should also be instructed to have the child rest, keep the foot elevated and use warm soaks

Stage 3 should be treated by removing the nail margin in a minor surgical outpatient procedure. Chronic ingrown toenails may require matrix ablation. This may be accomplished by surgical excision of a portion of the nail with ablation of the underlying matrix. Ablation is usually carried out by electrocautery of the underlying matrix. Caution must be used to avoid affecting tissue deep to the matrix. Enhanced results for treatment of chronic ingrown nails can be achieved by the addition of a chemical ablatant, phenol. Phenol is applied via a cotton-tipped applicator to the nail matrix to destroy the lateral portion of the matrix *(2 marks)*

Comment

Ingrown toenails (unguis incarnatus) are a common toenail problem of uncertain aetiology. Various causes include poorly fitting (tight) footwear, infection, improperly trimmed toenails, trauma and heredity. The great toe is the most commonly involved, with the lateral side is more commonly involved than the medial side. The underlying cause of this condition is a foreign body reaction. When the nailbed is compressed from the side, the edge of the nail penetrates the cuticle. The presence of keratinaceous material from the nail in the flesh of the toe sets up a foreign body reaction. The prevalence of ingrown nails has a reported male:female ratio of 3:1. The condition is observed in people of all ages but is most common in the second decade of life. Ingrown nails become much more common as children begin bearing weight on their feet and wearing shoes.

Answer 13

(a) Cauda equina syndrome   *(1 mark)*

(b) Disc herniation, spinal stenosis, spinal neoplasm
                                                    (3 marks)

(c) During development, the spinal cord and vertebral column grow at disproportionate rates, with the vertebral column growing more rapidly than the spinal cord. Spinal nerves exit the vertebral column at progressively more oblique angles as a result of the increasing distance between the spinal cord segments and the corresponding vertebrae. Lumbar and sacral nerves travel almost vertically down the spinal canal to reach their exiting foramen. The spinal cord tapers to an end near the first lumbar vertebra, forming the conus medullaris. The fibrous extension of the cord is the filum terminale. The bundle of nerve roots in the subarachnoid space distal to the conus medullaris is the cauda equina. Cauda equina syndrome refers to the simultaneous compression of multiple lumbosacral nerve roots below the level of the conus medullaris, resulting in a characteristic pattern of neuromuscular and urogenital symptoms   *(3 marks)*

(d) Nerve root ischaemia is partially responsible for the pain and decreased motor strength associated with the cauda equina syndrome. As a result, vasodilatory treatment can be useful in some patients

Treatment with lipoprostaglandin E_1 and its derivatives has been reported to be effective in increasing blood flow to the cauda equina region, reducing symptoms of pain and motor weakness. This treatment option should be reserved for patients with modest spinal stenosis and neurogenic claudication. No benefit has been reported in patients with more severe symptoms or patients with radicular symptoms

Patients with cauda equina syndrome secondary to infectious causes should receive appropriate antibiotic therapy. Patients with spinal neoplasms should be evaluated for the suitability of chemotherapy and radiotherapy

Caution should be used in any medical management of the cauda equina syndrome. Any patient with true cauda equina syndrome with symptoms of saddle anaesthesia and/or bilateral lower extremity weakness or loss of bowel or bladder control should undergo no more than 24 hours of initial medical management. If no relief of symptoms is achieved during this period, immediate surgical decompression is necessary to minimise the chances of permanent neurological injury

(3 marks)

Comment

Cauda equina syndrome is a serious neurological condition in which there is acute loss of function of the nerve roots of the spinal canal below the termination (conus) of the spinal cord. After the conus the canal contains a mass of nerves (the cauda equina), which travel caudally (towards the feet).

Any lesion that compresses or disturbs the function of the cauda equina may disable the nerves, although the most common is a central disc prolapse.

Other causes include protrusion of the vertebra into the canal if weakened by infection or tumour and an epidural abscess or haematoma.

Clinical features include weakness of the muscles innervated by the compressed roots (often paraplegia), sphincter weaknesses causing urinary retention and post-void residual incontinence as assessed by catheterisation after the patient has voided. In addition, there may be decreased rectal tone, sexual dysfunction, saddle anaesthesia, bilateral leg pain and weakness, and bilateral absence of ankle reflexes. Pain may, however, be wholly absent; the patient may complain only of lack of bladder control and of saddle anaesthesia, and may walk into the consulting room.

Diagnosis is usually confirmed by MRI or CT, depending on availability. If the cauda equina syndrome exists, early surgery is an option, depending on the aetiology discovered and the patient's candidacy for major spine surgery.

Answer 14

(a) The condition diagnosed by the neonatologist is termed 'congenital dislocation of the hip' and must be looked for during routine examination of newborn babies

Abduct both hips with knees and hips flexed to a right angle – the 'click' of reduction of a subluxated/dislocated hip is diagnostic

Subluxated hips are reduced and maintained in abduction with double nappies

Dislocated hips are reduced and held in an abduction splint (frog plaster spica) *(5 marks)*

(b) Joint laxity caused by unfavourable intrauterine posture, or genetic or placental hormonal factors

Dysplasia of the hip with deficient acetabulum and/or femoral head *(2 marks)*

(c) Treatment of established condition is difficult as a result of adaptive changes

Reduction of hip by closed or open method and maintained for at least 6 weeks

Any residual deformity is corrected by osteotomy. Acetabular dysplasia may require surgical correction at a later stage *(3 marks)*

Comment

Subluxated hips are not uncommon at birth (5–10 per 1000). Most reduce spontaneously soon after birth. Failure to diagnose and correct the dislocation before the child starts walking is negligent, because a good result is then difficult to achieve; osteoarthritis is a likely late complication.

Answer 15

(a) (i) Acute osteomyelitis of the radius/ulna   *(1 mark)*

(ii) Aspirate from area of maximal inflammation, send fluid for Gram staining and culture to identify the causative organism and its sensitivity

Raised WBC, ESR and anti-staphylococcal antibody titres   *(3 marks)*

(b) Cellulitis of the forearm
Acute suppurative arthritis of elbow
Sickle cell crisis
Gaucher's disease (pseudo-osteitis)   *(3 marks)*

(c) Analgesia and rehydration
Splint the forearm
Antibiotic therapy – initially broad spectrum, later sensitivity specific
Surgical drainage if abscess has formed   *(3 marks)*

Comment

Plain radiographs are of limited value during the first few days, because there is little or no radiological abnormality of the bone. By the end of the second week, periosteal new bone formation and metaphyseal mottling may be present – the classic radiological signs of pyogenic osteomyelitis. Treatment should commence immediately and not be delayed while waiting for these signs to appear. Cellulitis of the forearm may present an identical clinical picture and, in tropical climates, pyomyositis (inflammation of skeletal muscle) is caused by the same organisms. Accompanying septicaemia and fever may cause severe dehydration, and intravenous fluids may be required.

Answer 16

(a) (i) Childhood rickets *(1 mark)*

(ii) Radiology: thickening and widening of the epiphysis, cupping of the metaphysis, bowing of the diaphysis *(2 marks)*

(iii) Biochemistry: reduced serum Ca^{2+} and PO_4^{3-} ($Ca^{2+} \times PO_4^{3-} < 2.4$ diagnostic) Raised serum alkaline phosphatase *(2 marks)*

(b) (i) Underexposure to sunlight
Vitamin D deficiency from poor diet (or post-gastrectomy in adults) or malabsorption as a result of coeliac or pancreatic disease or small bowel surgery
Chronic liver or kidney disease *(3 marks)*

(ii) Dietary vitamin D supplementation with calcidol (vitamin D analogue) or calciferol (vitamin D_2) up to 40 000 units daily *(2 marks)*

Comment

In children, bowing of the tibia, if marked, may require the wearing of callipers to prevent further deformity and to restore normal alignment until new bone formation occurs. In adults the deficiency manifests as osteomalacia. The bones become deformed with an accompanying muscle weakness; correction of the deformities is by osteotomy.

Answer 17

(a) (i) Paget's disease of the spine (osteitis deformans) *(1 mark)*

(ii) Areas of osteoclastic activity with bone resorption, giving a radiological flame-shaped lesion along the shaft of bone

Adjacent areas of osteoblastic activity, with new bone formation, leading to radiological sclerosis and coarse trabeculation

Fibrovascular tissue is laid down in areas of bone
excavation   *(4 marks)*

(b) Skull enlargement, nerve compression and deafness
Pathological fracture
Osteoarthritis
Bone sarcoma   *(2 marks)*

(c) NSAIDs for bone and joint pain. Suppression of bone
turnover by calcitonin and bisphosphonates – effective
when the disease is in active phase:
Calcitonin decreases osteoclastic activity
Bisphosphonates reduce bone growth by binding to
hydroxyapatite crystals   *(3 marks)*

Comment
Most people with Paget's disease of the bone are asymptomatic,
and the disease comes to light during radiological investigation for
an unrelated condition. Surgery is reserved for complications of
pathological fractures (internal fixation with straightening of the
bone) and for nerve entrapment caused by severe spinal stenosis
(surgical decompression). Osteogenic sarcoma, if detected early,
may be resectable. A high-output cardiac failure and
hypercalcaemia may also be associated with the disease.

Answer 18

(a) (i) TB of the dorsal spine (Pott's disease of the
spine)   *(1 mark)*
(ii) Destruction of adjacent vertebral bodies by
caseation leads to collapse, producing spinal
angulation. The paravertebral abscess tracks down
deep to the psoas fascia and points in the
groin   *(2 marks)*

(b) Mantoux/Heaf skin test – positive
Raised ESR
Chest radiograph – evidence of primary lung lesion

Radiograph of entire spine – to detect distant occult lesions and to assess the degree of angulation and the number of vertebrae and disc spaces involved at the kyphosis

CT or MRI for evidence of impending cord compression

Needle aspiration of the groin abscess for histological and bacteriological confirmation   *(3 marks)*

(c) (i) Eradicate the disease with anti-tuberculous chemotherapy

Correct deformity and prevent spinal complications by drainage of paravertebral abscess and evacuation of infected/necrotic material

Correction of angulation with strut (rib) grafts and spinal fusion

Physiotherapy of the affected joints.

High protein diet   *(3 marks)*

(ii) Pott's paraplegia   *(1 mark)*

Comment

There is usually a long history of poor health and backache. Occasionally the patient may present with paraesthesiae and weakness of the legs. Spinal TB should be distinguished from other causes of vertebral destruction, i.e. pyogenic infections and malignant disease. Tumour metastases may cause vertebral body collapse but, in contrast to tuberculous spondylitis, the disc space is usually preserved.

Answer 19

(a) (i) Acute osteomyelitis of radius/ulna

Acute pyomyositis of flexor/extensor muscles

(2 marks)

(ii) The forearm is held still across the chest with the elbow flexed

Elbow and wrist movements are present, although the range of movements is restricted as a result of muscle spasm or bone pain   *(2 marks)*

(b) (i) *Staphylococcus aureus*
Streptococcus pyogenes
Haemophilus influenzae
Pneumococci
Salmonellae *(2 marks)*

(ii) Acute osteomyelitis and pyomyositis in the early phase respond well to antibiotic therapy

Sensitivity-specific agents are used once the organisms are isolated

Generally, however, intravenous cloxacillin 200 mg/kg daily in divided doses – followed, once the infection is under control, by oral flucloxacillin 100 mg daily

In penicillin allergies, a cephalosporin or fusidic acid and erythromycin may be substituted

Malnutrition must be treated with urgent dietary measures

No surgical measures are required in the early acute phase of either illness

Abscess formation requires drainage, and bone necrosis may occur in chronic osteomyelitis with involucrum formation, when surgical débridement is required *(4 marks)*

Comment

The aetiology of myositis and osteomyelitis is associated with a multitude of predisposing factors. Systemic bacterial infections, e.g. staphylococcal bacteraemia, may lead to seeding of the blood-borne organism in damaged or ischaemic muscle or bone. The presence of avitaminosis and malnutrition may lead to digestive enzyme deficiencies and chronic bowel infections with an overgrowth of intestinal organisms, namely *S. aureus*, being linked with muscle and bone infections in these children.

4

Neurosurgery

Answer 1

(a) Extradural (epidural) haematoma *(1 mark)*

(b) Most commonly a blow to the temple damages the middle meningeal artery. Arterial bleeding results in a rapid accumulation of blood in the extradural (epidural) space. *(1 mark)*

(c) Majority of extradural haematomas (EDHs) are located in the temporoparietal region where skull fractures cross the path of the middle meningeal artery or its dural branches. Expanding high-volume EDHs can produce a midline shift and subfalcine herniation of the brain. Compressed cerebral tissue can impinge on the third cranial nerve, resulting in ipsilateral pupillary dilation and contralateral hemiparesis or extensor motor response. EDHs are usually stable, attaining maximum size within minutes of injury. In nearly 10% of the patients EDHs can progress during first 24 hours rebleeding or continuous oozing. *(4 marks)*

(d) Early diagnosis and early surgery (if appropriate) are the key to a favourable outcome.
Drugs: Mannitol to reduce intracranial pressure.
Surgical: Burr holes or ideally craniotomy to evacuate haematoma. *(2 marks)*

(e) Outcome for extradural haematoma is often excellent if dealt with quickly, but less than a third of patients with best initial GCS of <8 will do well. Patients aged >65 have a worse prognosis. Mortality rate is 10-30%.

(2 marks)

Answer 2

(a) Acute subdural haematoma *(1 mark)*

(b) The usual mechanism to produce an acute subdural haematoma (SDH) is high-speed impact to the skull. This causes brain tissue to accelerate relative to a fixed dural structure, which, in turn, tears blood vessels. This mechanism also leads to associated contusions, brain oedema, and diffuse axonal injury. The ruptured blood vessel often is a vein connecting the cortical surface to the dural sinuses. Alternatively, a cortical vessel can be damaged by direct laceration. An acute SDH due to a ruptured cortical artery may be associated with only minor head injury, and no cerebral contusions may be associated. *(2 marks)*

(c) The clinical presentation of an acute SDH depends on the size of the haematoma and the degree of any associated parenchymal brain injury.
All patients with traumatic brain injury should be evaluated using the Glasgow Coma Score (GCS). Common neurological findings include (1) altered level of consciousness, (2) a dilated pupil ipsilateral to the haematoma, (3) failure of the ipsilateral pupil to react to light, and (4) hemiparesis contralateral to the haematoma.
The patient should be examined for related injuries such as spinal cord injury or long bone fractures.

(4 marks)

  (d) Small acute SDHs less than 5 mm thick on axial CT images, without sufficient mass effect to cause midline shift or neurological signs, can be followed clinically with serial imaging.

       Emergent medical treatment of an acute SDH causing impending transtentorial herniation is the bolus administration of mannitol (in the patient who is adequately fluid resuscitated with an adequate blood pressure). Surgical evacuation of the lesion is the definitive treatment and should not be delayed.

(3 marks)

Answer 3

  (a) Right-sided cerebral abscess: chronic infections from the paranasal sinuses produce a thrombophlebitis that may extend into the cranium through the cribriform plate and infect the subdural space, resulting in an abscess   *(3 marks)*

  (b) CT or MRI, which may be contrast enhanced   *(2 marks)*

  (c) Aspiration of the abscess under stereotactic control and intravenous antibiotic therapy guided by the culture and sensitivity result of the aspirated pus; if the abscess is large or multi-loculated, drainage through a craniotomy may provide access for breakdown of loculi and irrigation of the subdural space   *(5 marks)*

Comment

Intracranial abscesses may arise extradurally, subdurally or within the brain. Scalp infection or an open skull fracture may directly infect the extradural space, whereas a thrombophlebitis of the cerebral veins from a middle-ear or sinus infection may infect the subdural space. This is more likely in an immunocompromised patient.

Answer 4

    (a)   Astrocytoma
            Ependymoma
            Oligodendroglioma
            Medulloblastoma   *(2 marks)*

    (b)   Burr hole biopsy under ultrasound guidance   *(2 marks)*

    (c)   Surgical excision: complete, in circumscribed/accessible
            tumours; partial, in extensive/inaccessible tumours
            Adjuvant therapy: radiotherapy/chemotherapy to treat
            residual disease
            Aim: to achieve a cure, alleviate symptoms
            and restore neurological function   *(6 marks)*

Comment

An anatomical diagnosis of a brain tumour is usually made on
clinical and imaging evidence; this determines surgical access and
potential complications from involvement of adjacent structures.
Histological verification is usually by open biopsy and is not always
feasible because of the hazards of this procedure. Surgical excision
may be limited to avoid neurological sequelae, but adjuvant
radiotherapy or chemotherapy may give good palliation, depending
on the tumour type and its malignant potential.

Answer 5

    (a)   Electroencephalogram (EEG)
            MRI of the brain
            Videotelemetry of cerebral activity   *(3 marks)*

    (b)   Failure of an adequate trial of anticonvulsant drug
            therapy increased to the highest tolerable dosage
            Surgical access with localisation of the seizure focus
            Evidence that surgery would improve overall
            quality of life
            Absence of psychiatric illness   *(4 marks)*

CHAPTER 4 – ANSWERS

(c) Patients (and carers) should be informed of the following:

Postoperative psychological morbidity – usually transient; rarely, personality changes may persist

Seizures may not be completely abolished after surgery; however, there is a reduction in their frequency and duration

Coexisting personality disorders would not be improved but post-ictal psychosis may respond favourably   *(3 marks)*

Comment

The clinical examination of patients with epilepsy is frequently normal. Focal lesions producing seizures are often the result of ischaemic episodes, haemorrhage or tumours. EEG and videotelemetric monitoring of brain activity localises the source of abnormal neuronal activity and, together with cerebral imaging, assists in planning surgical treatment. The principle of seizure surgery is excision of an identifiable focal cerebral lesion; intraoperative electrocorticography and cortical stimulation under local anaesthesia identify the limits of surgical excision, particularly when involving the dominant cerebral hemisphere.

Answer 6

(a) (i) Infantile hydrocephalus   *(1 mark)*

    (ii) Tense anterior fontanelle
'Cracked pot' sound on percussion
Transillumination of cranial cavity
'Setting sun' appearance of the eyes
Thin scalp with dilated veins
Abnormally large skull compared with
normal growth charts   *(2 marks)*

    (iii) CT or MRI head scan   *(1 mark)*

(b) (i) Stenosis of the aqueduct of Sylvius
causes a sustained rise in ICP   *(1 mark)*

    (ii) Spina bifida
Meningomyelocele   *(2 marks)*

(c) Cerebrospinal fluid (CSF) shunt with a one-way valve between the lateral ventricle and right atrium or peritoneum *(3 marks)*

Comment

Hydrocephalus may be diagnosed prenatally by ultrasonography. Treatment of infantile hydrocephalus is by shunting, except in the rare, chronic (arrested) hydrocephalus, where the CSF pressure has returned to normal. These children require careful neurological follow-up to detect any deterioration. After shunting, ventricular size can be monitored by ultrasonography through the open anterior fontanelle. The overall prognosis is poor, with a third dying and a third achieving a semblance of normality by the age of 10 years.

Answer 7

(a) (i) Intracranial space-occupying lesion *(1 mark)*
(ii) Raised ICP as a result of a tumour mass with or without obstruction of CSF circulation
Fits may be the result of a mass effect or pressure on motor pathways *(3 marks)*

(b) (i) Cranial CT or MRI
Cerebral angiography *(2 marks)*
(ii) Herniation of the brain stem into the foramen magnum (coning) *(1 mark)*

(c) Benign tumours:
Meningioma
Acoustic neuroma
Haemangioblastoma
Epidermoid and dermoid cysts
Colloid cyst of the third ventricle
Malignant tumours:
Neuroepithelial tumour
Germ cell tumour
Lymphomas and leukaemias
Metastatic tumours *(3 marks)*

Comment

Epilepsy is the most frequent initial symptom of a glioma or meningioma. Headaches that are present on waking, changing posture, coughing or straining, or of unusual intensity, and occurring in those not previously prone to headaches merit CT. Changes in personality, cognitive function and memory are also features suggestive of a brain tumour.

Answer 8

(a) (i)   A subarachnoid haemorrhage caused by a ruptured cerebral aneurysm or arteriovenous malformation   *(2 marks)*

(ii)   Increasing drowsiness leading to stupor and coma; simultaneously mild focal neurological deficit may progress to moderate and then severe hemiparesis, leading to decerebrate rigidity   *(3 marks)*

(b) (i)   CT or MRI head scan   *(1 mark)*

(ii)   Xanthochromia and sterile CSF   *(1 mark)*

(c)   Medical measures:
  • Bedrest, sedation and adequate analgesia
  • Treat hypertension when present
  • Maintain fluid and electrolyte balance
  • Surgery: control bleeding by clipping the aneurysm or feeding vessels to arteriovenous malformation
                                                                    (3 marks)

Comment

A sudden bleed into the subarachnoid space is soon followed by cerebral oedema and a raised ICP. Lumbar puncture in these circumstances may cause coning; if, however, fulminant meningitis cannot be ruled out, it may be carried out once the ICP stabilises. Nimodipine, a calcium-channel blocker, reduces the incidence of infarction and ischaemic deficits when administered soon after the haemorrhage.

Answer 9

(a) (i)   Right hemiparesis/hemiplegia
            Dysphasia
            Right-sided sensory disturbance   *(2 marks)*

     (ii) Hypertension, polycythaemia, diabetes mellitus,
            alcoholism, smoking, hyperlipidaemia
            Atrial fibrillation or valvular heart
            disease   *(2 marks)*

(b) Cranial CT or MRI to evaluate the extent of cerebral
     infarction and oedema, and presence of an intracranial
     haemorrhage

     Maintain airway

     Anticoagulation if thrombosis/embolism diagnosed
     with four hours of outset, with intravenous heparin
     40 000 units/24 h

     Lower raised ICP: positive pressure ventilation with 5%
     P_{CO_2}

     Reduce cerebral oedema: mannitol infusion and/or
     corticosteroid therapy

     Maintain fluid, electrolyte and acid–base
     balance   *(6 marks)*

Comment

Investigations should be directed towards categorising the vascular
event as a guide to prognosis. Surgical measures for improving
cerebral perfusion or for cerebral decompression do not generally
improve prognosis. Surgery may have a role in preventing
subsequent stroke in those who survive the initial event.

Answer 10

(a) A history of a prodromal period with malaise, fever and
     listlessness
     Clinical features of an underlying source of infection
     Focal neurological signs (including epileptic fits)
     Change in level of consciousness, i.e. drowsiness
     or irritability   *(3 marks)*

CHAPTER 4 – ANSWERS

(b) (i) Streptococci
         Staphylococcus aureus
         Proteus spp.
         Bacteroides fragilis
         E. coli
         Haemophilus influenzae   (2 marks)
    (ii) Bronchitis/pneumonia
         Otitis media
         Sinus infection
         Gastroenteritis   (2 marks)

(c) Correct fluid and electrolyte balance
    Sedation
    Initially broad-spectrum antimicrobial therapy, then
    specific agent(s) once pus culture and sensitivity are
    available
    Surgical aspiration or excision   (3 marks)

Comment

A brain abscess is a mass lesion producing focal neurological signs
and must be distinguished from meningitis. Lumbar puncture is
contraindicated as a result of the danger of tentorial herniation.

Antibiotic therapy: the initial choice of antibiotic before culture
results are available will depend on the probable cause of the
abscess and the Gram stain.

Aspiration of an abscess may be performed using CT-guided
stereotaxis. Aspiration may need to be repeated with a CT follow-
up. Surgical excision is indicated:

- For persistent reaccumulation despite repeated aspirations
- If the abscess is not accessible for aspiration
- In the presence of a fibrous capsule surrounding the abscess,
  preventing collapse on aspiration.

Answer 11

(a) Cervical cord lesion causing compression: extradural abscess; metastatic tumours; intradural tumours, e.g. meningioma, schwannoma; intramedullary tumours, e.g. gliomas
Spinal lesions causing compression: cervical spondylolisthesis/spondylitis; intervertebral disc prolapse; infections of vertebral body (e.g. Pott's disease) *(3 marks)*

(b) Muscle wasting and lower motor neuron weakness, with sensory disturbance of nerve roots C5–T1 *(3 marks)*

(c) (i) Plain cervical spine radiographs
Myelography
CT (with intrathecal contrast) or MRI *(2 marks)*
(ii) Mild symptoms caused by degenerative lesions of the spine respond well to analgesics, rest, physiotherapy and wearing of a collar
Surgical decompression of the cervical cord is required occasionally as an emergency for progressive neurological signs
Radiotherapy with corticosteroids is indicated for malignant cord compression *(2 marks)*

Comment

A feature of spinal cord compression is local and radicular pain that predates sensory and motor disturbances. Urinary sphincter disturbances may also be present. The tingling, or 'electric shock', sensation on flexion/extension of the neck (L'Hermitte's sign) is diagnostic. Metastatic tumour deposits are from the lung, breast, kidney and prostate. Tumours of the reticuloendothelial system also metastasise to the spine. Urgent surgery is required for progressive neurological signs to avoid permanent disability. Palliative radiotherapy in malignant disease relieves pain and may produce a partial remission of weakness. It may be as effective in metastatic disease as surgical decompression.

CHAPTER 4 – ANSWERS

5 | Skin, Eyes and ENT

Answer 1

(a) Cancrum oris (noma) *(2 marks)*

(b) Protein–calorie malnutrition
Chronic anaemia (hookworm infestation)
Measles
Poor oral hygiene during the period of tooth
eruption *(3 marks)*

(c) Parenteral broad-spectrum antibiotic therapy
Nasogastric feeding of high protein–calorie diet
Antiseptic mouthwash and wound irrigation
Closure of defect after healing with a cutaneous
pedicled flap transfer *(5 marks)*

Comment

This is a necrotising stomatitis or a severe form of ulcerative gingivitis arising from the gums and spreading to the mandible and the cheek, resulting in a gaping hole in the side of the face; the child is at risk of developing overwhelming sepsis. The infection must, therefore, be treated urgently with intravenous penicillin and metronidazole with frequent wound irrigation. The accompanying malnutrition must be corrected; a blood transfusion may be required to correct severe anaemia. Surgery is deferred until healing and involves excision of the contracture (which produces trismus) and a pedicled skin flap closure of the defect.

Answer 2

(a) (i) Burkitt's lymphoma *(2 marks)*
    (ii) Plain radiology of the facial bones
         Intraoral biopsy *(2 marks)*

(b) Affects pre-adolescent children confined to the
    equatorial belt of 4° latitude, which includes the
    tropical rain forest
    The Epstein–Barr virus
    Chronic malnutrition *(3 marks)*

(c) Oral cyclophosphamide alone or in
    combination *(3 marks)*

Comment

This is a childhood tumour confined to a tropical geographical
belt, implicating environmental factors in its causation. It was first
studied in children in equatorial Africa, but is also found in New
Guinea and Central America. The tumour arises from the jaw,
close to the alveolar margin, with radiological signs of its
disruption. The response to cyclophosphamide is usually rapid
and combination chemotherapy produces long-term remission.

Answer 3

(a) Squamous carcinoma (Marjolin's ulcer)
    An ulcerating lesion, minimally tender, with an
    indurated base and everted edges; surrounded by thin
    or hypertrophic scar tissue; popliteal or groin
    lymphadenopathy; may be palpable *(4 marks)*

(b) Incisional biopsy from edge of ulcer *(2 marks)*

(c) Excision of the ulcer with a 2 cm clear margin
    extending down to the fascia and split-skin or pedicled
    flap grafting
    Block dissection of palpable groin nodes or if found to
    contain tumour after sentinel node biopsy *(4 marks)*

Comment

When a squamous carcinoma develops in a cutaneous scar, it is usually as a result of poor healing or chronic irritation. It differs from other skin cancers in that it is relatively painless and grows slowly over a prolonged period. Distant metastases are delayed as a result of the paucity of blood supply and lymphatic drainage in scar tissue. During surgical excision it is advisable to include as much of the surrounding scar tissue as possible.

Answer 4

(a) Basal cell carcinoma   *(1 mark)*

(b) The three conditions which may be considered in the differential diagnosis of basal cell carcinoma include:
1.   Squamous cell carcinoma
2.   Keratoacanthoma
3.   Actinic keratosis   *(3 marks)*

(c) Biopsy is required to confirm the diagnosis and to identify histologic subtype of the basal cell carcinoma (BCC). Shave or punch biopsy is usually performed. Additional workup is rarely necessary, unless a genetic disorder is suspected.   *(3 marks)*

(d) The treatment of basal cell carcinoma may be discussed under two headings.
Medical Care: Local therapy with chemotherapeutic and immune-modulating agents is useful in some cases of multiple or recurrent small and superficial BCC.
Surgical Care: The goal of surgical treatment of BCC is to destroy or remove the tumour so that no malignant tissue is allowed to proliferate further. The most common surgical methods are curettage, excision with margin examination, Mohs micrographic surgery, and radiotherapy. Cryotherapy is sometimes used to treat these tumours.   *(3 marks)*

Answer 5

(a) (i) The lesion: the edge, base, floor and surrounding skin

Regional lymph nodes *(1 mark)*

(ii) Malignant melanoma *(1 mark)*

(iii) Depth of invasion is measured from the top of the granular layer of the epidermis to the deepest melanoma cell in the dermis

Tumour thickness < 0.76 mm has a favourable prognosis *(2 marks)*

(b) Wide local excision down to deep fascia

If histologically malignant:

- Sentinel node biopsy
- Radiotherapy with/without nodal clearance and/or chemotherapy based on histological staging or distant spread *(3 marks)*

(c) Protection from sun by clothing and wide-brimmed hats

Apply sunscreen lotions containing skin protection factors and limit time of exposure *(3 marks)*

Comment

Malignant change in a pre-existing naevus is difficult to assess because there is uncertainty about whether melanomas always arise from pigmented moles. However, a change in size, itchiness or bleeding should arouse suspicion. Delayed or missed diagnosis may result in dissemination, although it is unclear if this occurs during the radial or vertical growth phases. Diagnosis is by histological examination of the whole lesion and incisional biopsy is, therefore, ill-advised.

Answer 6

(a) BCC
Malignant melanoma
Squamous cell carcinoma   *(3 marks)*

(b) Excision for histological confirmation with adequate
surrounding clearance. Plastic surgery may be required
to close the defect. Cryosurgery or curettage and
cautery is suited for small lesions. Radiotherapy for
BCC is an option when surgery is inappropriate for
lesions close to the eye   *(4 marks)*

(c) (i) UV light on certain skin types produces
dysplasia of epidermal cell layers leading to
actinic keratosis; this may progress to
invasive tumours   *(2 marks)*
(ii) Wearing protective clothing and headgear;
limit exposure to direct sunlight and apply
sunscreen lotions during exposure   *(1 mark)*

Comment

The choice of treatment for facial lesions is based on the size of the
tumour and the physical state of the patient, as well as cosmetic
considerations. In general, surgery is preferred for those lesions
that can be totally excised and the skin closed with minimal
cosmetic disfigurement.

Interestingly, most melanomas occur on skin that is only
intermittently exposed to the sun; individuals with higher
continuous exposure have lower rates than those exposed
intermittently and, curiously, the use of sunscreens may increase
rather than decrease the melanoma risk. Most dysplastic lesions do
not progress to skin malignancy; some may regress with time.

Answer 7

(a) Occlusion of central retinal artery or vein
Ischaemic optic neuropathy
Retinal detachment
Vitreous haemorrhage
Temporal arteritis
Hysterical blindness
Macular lesions   *(4 marks)*

(b) Atherosclerosis
Hypertension
Diabetes mellitus   *(3 marks)*

(c) Any lesion involving the optic chiasma,
including ischaemic infarction
Hysterical blindness   *(3 marks)*

Comment

The fundus in central retinal artery occlusion is creamy white as a result of an infarcted retina, except over the macula, which is visible as 'the cherry-red spot'. In ischaemic optic neuropathy (caused by temporal arteritis), a pale and swollen optic disc is present; in retinal detachment the opaque retina obscures the normal choroidal red glow, and instead there is a grey, rippled reflex.

Answer 8

(a) Conjunctivitis
Episcleritis and scleritis
Keratitis
Uveitis   *(2 marks)*

(b) Look for a foreign body in the conjunctiva
Pupillary reflexes to light
Slitlamp examination of iris and lens
Fundoscopic examination of the retina
Fluorescein stain for corneal abrasions/
ulcer   *(4 marks)*

(c) Retinoblastoma: enucleation with chemo-
and/or radiotherapy   *(4 marks)*

Comment

Three major causes of red eye in adults are: iritis, keratitis and acute angle-closure (acute) glaucoma. Signs on slitlamp examination are: ciliary injection and white deposits on the corneal surface in iritis; a broken corneal epithelium in keratitis; and a hazy cornea with a shallow anterior chamber and a dilated pupil in acute glaucoma.

Answer 9

(a) (i) Acute orbital cellulites   *(1 mark)*

    (ii) Conjunctival and nasopharyngeal swabs for culture and sensitivity
Aerobic and anaerobic blood cultures
AP and lateral radiographs of paranasal sinuses and orbit   *(2 marks)*

(b) (i) Broad-spectrum intravenous antibiotic therapy, changing if required to sensitivity specific
Intravenous rehydration
Pain relief and sedation as required   *(2 marks)*

    (ii) Place on a pulse and temperature chart
Test visual acuity and pupillary reaction twice daily and examine the optic disc daily
Serial ultrasonography or CT to detect early signs of subperiosteal abscess formation   *(2 marks)*

(c) (i) Surgical drainage and/or excision of the ethmoidal sinus, with drainage of frontal and sphenoidal sinuses   *(2 marks)*

    (ii) Cavernous sinus thrombosis, which may lead to a brain abscess   *(1 mark)*

Comment

Acute orbital cellulitis is the most common cause of exophthalmos in children and usually spreads from an infected ethmoid sinus. Preseptal cellulitis, which is a common complication of acute sinusitis, may spread to the orbit, because orbital septa are not well developed in children. After recovery on antibiotic therapy, the underlying paranasal sinusitis must be treated to prevent recurrences. Orbital surgical exploration is required if the infection cannot be controlled by antibiotics, with the danger of the infection spreading to the globe (panophthalmitis).

Answer 10

(a) (i) Blow-out fracture of the orbital floor   *(1 mark)*

     (ii) A hard object > 5 cm in diameter striking the orbit causes a sudden increase in intraorbital pressure, which produces orbital floor fracture   *(2 marks)*

(b) (i) Infraorbital nerve injury causes anaesthesia involving the lower eyelid, cheek, side of nose, upper lip and teeth. Diplopia, when present, is typically vertical in both up- and downgaze, and is caused by tethering of extraocular muscles to the fracture line. Enophthalmos may be present initially or may appear later as the periorbital oedema subsides and the eyeball sinks into the fractured floor   *(3 marks)*

     (ii) Plain orbital radiographs (Waters' view) CT scan of orbit (axial and coronal sections)   *(1 mark)*

(c) Small cracks in the orbital floor without diplopia require no treatment. Fractures of less than 50% of the floor, with improving diplopia, require no treatment unless enophthalmos is more than 2 mm. Fractures of over 50% of the floor, with persistent diplopia, should be repaired within 2 weeks of injury   *(3 marks)*

Comment

Despite the invariable presence of conjunctival ecchymosis and chemosis, orbital injuries rarely cause ocular damage. Surgical treatment of orbital floor fractures entails freeing the entrapped tissue and covering the defect with a plastic plate. Orbital margins offer little protection to small missiles, such as squash balls and shuttlecocks, that may impact directly on to the eyeball and cause serious ocular injury.

Answer 11

(a) (i)   Acute recurrent tonsillitis   *(2 marks)*
       (ii) Adenoidal hypertrophy   *(2 marks)*

(b) Palpable cervical lymph node (tonsillar node) largyngoscopy; tonsils swollen, inflamed and indurated; pus may be expressed from the tonsillar crypts   *(3 marks)*

(c) Tonsillectomy and adenoidectomy under antibiotic cover   *(3 marks)*

Comment

Adenoidal hypertrophy is a frequent accompaniment of tonsillar hypertrophy from recurrent bacterial infection, and is implicated in obstructive sleep apnoea syndrome and sudden infant death syndrome. The indications for tonsillectomy are recurrent attacks of tonsillitis (more than three episodes/year), peritonsillar abscess (quinsy) and chronic tonsillitis, particularly if associated with respiratory, cardiac, renal or rheumatic illness. Indications for adenoidectomy are recurrent middle-ear infection, postnasal obstruction or discharge, or recurrent sinusitis

Answer 12

(a) Chronic laryngitis caused by vocal abuse, tobacco use or myxoedema
Laryngeal polyps, nodules, granulomas and papillomas   *(2 marks)*

(b) Indirect laryngoscopy by use of a laryngeal mirror with or without pharyngeal anaesthetic spray
Fibreoptic laryngoscopy via nostril with topical anaesthetic spray
Direct laryngoscopy under general anaesthetic (e.g. in children)   *(4 marks)*

(c) Radiotherapy for most early lesions – with a cure rate of 90%
Laser beam surgical excision of early lesions is also curative
For extensive vocal fold carcinomas, a partial or total laryngectomy may be performed in conjunction with a neck dissection for nodal involvement
Total laryngectomy requires a tracheostomy and oesophageal voice training *(4 marks)*

Comment

Laryngeal nodules, a specific and localised form of chronic laryngitis, are found in professional voice users (singer's nodules) and in children (screamer's nodules). Juvenile papillomas must be excluded in hoarseness in children; they are caused by the human papilloma virus.

Carcinomas may present above (supraglottic) or below (infraglottic) the vocal folds. They have a worse prognosis than glottic tumours, because hoarseness is a late symptom and diagnosis is delayed until the vocal fold is involved; the greater vascularity and lymphatic drainage above and below the cord predispose to earlier metastases.

Answer 13

(a) Epistaxis *(1 mark)*

(b) Epistaxis is classified on the basis of the primary bleeding site as anterior or posterior. Haemorrhage is most commonly anterior, originating from the nasal septum. A common source of anterior epistaxis is the Kiesselbach plexus, an anastomotic network of vessels on the anterior portion of the nasal septum. Anterior bleeding may also originate anterior to the inferior turbinate. Posterior hemorrhage originates from branches of the sphenopalatine artery in the posterior nasal cavity or nasopharynx. *(2 marks)*

(c)   The causes for epistaxis include:
1.   Local trauma (ie, nose picking) is the most common cause, followed by facial trauma, foreign bodies, nasal or sinus infections, and prolonged inhalation of dry air. A disturbance of normal nasal airflow, as occurs in a deviated nasal septum, may also be a cause of epistaxis.
2.   Iatrogenic causes include nasogastric and nasotracheal intubation.
3.   Children usually present with epistaxis due to local irritation or recent upper respiratory infection.

(3 marks)

(d)   The management of epistaxis can be outlined as follows:
- Continuous local pressure for at least 10 minutes.
- Insert pledgets soaked with an anaesthetic-vasoconstrictor solution into the nasal cavity to anesthetise and shrink nasal mucosa.
- Chemical cautery after the application of adequate topical anesthesia.
- Address the patient's airway, breathing, and circulation (ABCs) in case of severe epistaxis.
- Severe epistaxis may require endotracheal intubation.
- Rapid control of massive bleeding is best secured with an epistaxis balloon or Foley catheter.
- Volume replacement in case of significant blood loss.
- Nasal packing if all else fails.   *(4 marks)*

Answer 14

(a)   Chronic suppurative otitis media with cholesteatoma

(2 marks)

(b)   Chronic otitis media is associated with the following conditions:
- Poor socioeconomic status
- Overcrowding
- Poor nutrition
- Poor hygiene
- Infectious diseases (eg, measles)

The disorder is more prevalent in some specific populations, such as Eskimos and American Indians, as well as in people with cleft palates.

Adenoid hypertrophy and chronic sinusitis also contribute to the development of chronic suppurative otitis media. *(2 marks)*

(c) Chronic otitis media develops after longstanding inflammation of the middle ear cleft. There are likely a number of reasons for the inflammation, including acute otitis media, perforation of the tympanic membrane and eustachian tube dysfunction. The exposure to chronic inflammatory mediators leads to weakening of the tympanic membrane while causing mucosal oedema. Eventually eustachian tube dysfunction leads to negative middle ear pressure that causes tympanic membrane retraction and perforation. Longstanding negative pressure can damage surrounding bone and ossicles, leading to cholesteatoma or loss of ossicular continuity.

(3 marks)

(d) General indications for surgery are as follows:
- Perforation that persists beyond 6 weeks
- Otorrhea (ear discharge) that persists for longer than 6 weeks despite antibiotic use
- Cholesteatoma formation
- Radiographic evidence of chronic mastoiditis, such as coalescent mastoiditis
- Conductive hearing loss *(3 marks)*

Answer 15

(a) (i) Conductive deafness caused by secretory otitis media is a result of eustachian tube dysfunction *(2 marks)*

(ii) Predisposition:
Acute otitis media
Adenoidal inflammation
Postnasal space neoplasm
Barotrauma *(2 marks)*

(b) There is reduced mobility of the eardrum, with hyperaemia
The middle-ear effusion may alter in composition and appear golden-brown or blue
Occasionally bubbles may be seen through the drum
A retracted drum with prominent malleus and occasional vesicles   *(2 marks)*

(c) Myringotomy: aspiration of fluid under a general anaesthetic if troublesome symptoms persist for over 3 months
Insertion of a grommet (a tiny flanged Teflon tube) into the drum is frequently required to avoid recurrence of middle ear fluid
An anterior or inferior radial myringotomy incision is used to insert the grommet   *(4 marks)*

Comment

Secretory otitis media may settle spontaneously. Nasal vasoconstrictor drops with an oral decongestant may assist 'recovery' when there is an associated upper respiratory tract infection. A marked and persistent hearing loss that interferes with schooling necessitates surgery. This may involve the insertion of a grommet to drain and ventilate the middle ear. The grommet usually extrudes spontaneously 6–18 months after insertion. If normal eustachian tube function has not returned and secretory otitis media recurs, the grommet is replaced.

6

Endocrinology and Breast

Answer 1

(a) (i) Goitre
Parathyroid adenoma
Thyroglossal cyst
Cervical lymphadenopathy
Dermoid and epidermal cysts
Branchial cysts and carotid body tumours are
located to the side of the neck   *(2 marks)*

(ii) Thyroid and parathyroid glands: move with
swelling
Thyroglossal cyst: lies over hyoid bone and moves
up on tongue protrusion
Branchial cyst: lies near angle of mandible
Lymph nodes: usually lateral to the
midline and may be multiple   *(2 marks)*

(b) Neck and thoracic inlet views
Ultrasonography, radio-isotope scan
Thyroid function tests, serum Ca^{2+}
Fine-needle aspiration cytology (FNAC)   *(2 marks)*

(c) Thyroid cancer or when malignancy cannot be
excluded
Dyspnoea caused by tracheal deviation/compression
Toxicity non-responsiveness to anti-thyroid agents
Retrosternal extension
Cosmetic considerations   *(4 marks)*

Comment

A swelling located over the thyroid cartilage is almost invariably a goitre and requires functional assessment. Branchial and thyroglossal cysts require excision because they are liable to become infected and symptomatic. Enlarged cervical lymph nodes are caused by a host of local and systemic factors, and node biopsy may be required to assess in diagnosis or treatment. Thyroid cancers are treated surgically by total or near-total thyroidectomy, except for some anaplastic tumours and lymphomas. The latter respond well to chemotherapy, whereas, in the former, the response to any form of treatment is poor.

Answer 2

(a) (i)   Thyrotoxicosis   *(1 mark)*

 (ii) Proptosis, lid lag, lid retraction
       Fine tremor, rapid sleeping pulse
       Thyroid bruit, functional systolic murmur
       Atrial fibrillation   *(3 marks)*

(b) TSH (thyroid-stimulating hormone), T_3 (tri-iodothyronine), T_4 (thyroxine)
     ^{131}I-labelled thyroid scan   *(3 marks)*

(c) Inpatient monitoring of pulse, BP and respiration
     Anti-thyroid drugs, e.g. carbimazole
     Anti-arrhythmic agents, e.g. propranolol
     Night sedation, e.g. nitrazepam
     Subtotal thyroidectomy when the patient is euthyroid
     Lugol's iodine administered for a few days
     preoperatively   *(3 marks)*

Comment

Subtotal thyroidectomy is the treatment of choice for thyrotoxicosis; anti-thyroid agents may lead to recurrence of symptoms after cessation of treatment; radio-iodine therapy leads to hypothyroidism over a period of time and is contraindicated in young adults. In the presence of eye signs the condition is referred to as Graves' disease. Eye signs rarely respond to medical measures or subtotal thyroidectomy. Orbital decompression or tarsorraphy may be required for cosmetic purposes and occasionally for conjunctivitis and chemosis.

Answer 3

(a) Texture and firmness of goitre
Retrosternal extension
Tenderness on palpation
Presence of palpable neck nodes suggests papillary, medullary or anaplastic tumours
Palpable bony lesions suggest follicular or anaplastic carcinoma   *(3 marks)*

(b) Thyroid malignancy invading the larynx or the recurrent laryngeal nerve causing vocal fold palsy
Indirect laryngoscopy   *(2 marks)*

(c) (i) Ultrasound scan of the thyroid with guided FNAC or core needle biopsy
Radiograph of neck and thoracic inlet
^{131}I-uptake thyroid scan; selenium–methionine scan   *(3 marks)*

(ii) Poor or no uptake of the isotope ^{131}I in a discrete area suggests absence of functional thyroid tissue. This may represent a cystic lesion or a solid lesion, e.g. a follicular adenoma or a carcinoma   *(2 marks)*

Comment
Papillary carcinomas account for 60% of all thyroid malignancies and have a good prognosis, despite nodal recurrence. Lymphatic spread also occurs in medullary (C-cell) and anaplastic carcinomas, but blood-borne spread is common and the prognosis poor. Calcitonin is produced by medullary tumours and is used as a tumour marker to detect recurrence following total thyroidectomy.

Answer 4

(a) Ca^{2+} and phosphate are lost from bone as a result of loss of renal tubular reabsorption, leading to osteoporosis *(3 marks)*

(b) Fall in serum Ca^{2+} as a result of urinary loss stimulates PTH secretion and, if sustained, leads to parathyroid hyperplasia *(3 marks)*

(c) Remove all parathyroid glands and place the patient on long-term-cholecalciferol (vitamin D analogue) therapy *(4 marks)*

Comment

In primary hyperparathyroidism the increased PTH production is the result of primary hyperplasia, an adenoma or, rarely, a carcinoma of the parathyroid. Treatment consists of removal of all four glands, when hyperplasic, with possible reimplantation of a portion of one gland in a surgically accessible site. When removing a functional adenoma or a carcinoma the other glands are usually hypoplastic and do not require removal.

Secondary hyperparathyroidism is caused by a sustained low serum Ca^{2+} level from any cause. Re-establishing normal serum Ca^{2+} should lead to resolution of the hyperplastic state, although this is uncommon in chronic renal failure.

In tertiary hyperparathyroidism PTH production becomes independent of serum Ca^{2+} levels, and the glands become autonomous, leading to hypercalcaemic states. Total parathyroidectomy and vitamin D analogue administration bring about homoeostasis.

Answer 5

(a) (i) Phaeochromocytoma *(1 mark)*

(ii) Serum and urinary norepinephrine and/or epinephrine levels are elevated *(2 marks)*

(b) (i) The catecholamines secreted by the tumour
produce cardiovascular instability, i.e.
hypertension and cardiac arrhythmias *(2 marks)*

(ii) β-blockade by phenoxybenzamine (20–80 mg
daily in divided doses) lowers the BP
β-blockade by propranolol (120–140 mg daily in
divided doses) converts cardiac irregularities
to sinus rhythm *(3 marks)*

(iii) Adrenalectomy *(2 marks)*

Comment

Phaeochromocytomas are neuroectodermal tumours of the
sympathetic chain, 90% of which arise in the adrenal gland and the
remainder elsewhere along the chain. Most tumours release both
epinephrine and norepinephrine but large tumours produce only
norepinephrine. Scanning with[^{131}I] or [^{132}I]
metaiodobenzylguanidine (MIBG) produces specific uptake in sites
of sympathetic activity and is used for diagnostic confirmation.
Adrenal surgery must be supported by α- and β-blockade (the
former preceding the latter), along with whole-blood transfusion as
required to re-expand the contracted intravascular volume.

Answer 6

(a) (i) Cushing's disease or syndrome *(1 mark)*

(ii) Dexamethasone suppression test *(1 mark)*

(b) (i) Pituitary gland or adrenal gland *(1 mark)*

(ii) High-resolution CT with intravenous
contrast or MRI *(1 mark)*

(iii) Pituitary gland:
 • Gigantism or acromegaly
 • Hyperprolactinaemic syndrome
 • Thyrotoxicosis
 • Adrenal gland:
 • Phaeochromocytoma
 • Conn's syndrome
 • Addison's disease *(3 marks)*

CHAPTER 6 – ANSWERS

(c)   Medical treatment with anti-secretory drugs
Surgical removal of pituitary tumour by trans-
sphenoidal hypophysectomy
Radiotherapy if surgical excision is
incomplete   *(3 marks)*

Comment

Cushing's disease is caused by an adrenocorticotrophin (ACTH)-
secreting pituitary tumour, resulting in bilateral adrenocortical
hyperplasia and secretion of adrenal corticosteroids. Cushing's
syndrome is the result of an adrenal tumour or a cortisol-secreting
ectopic source, such as a bronchial carcinoma. The diagnosis of
Cushing's disease is based on a failure of the pituitary source of
ACTH to be suppressed by dexamethasone. Corticotrophin-
releasing hormone given to those with a pituitary source of ACTH
results in a normal or exaggerated corticotrophin or cortisol
response, but adrenal tumours or ectopic sources of ACTH do not
respond.

Answer 7

(a)   (i)   Express nipple discharge
Thickening/eczema of nipple; peau d'orange
Palpable lesion underlying the nipple
areolar complex   *(2 marks)*
(ii)   Supraclavicular nodes
Axillary nodes
Liver enlargement
Contralateral breast   *(2 marks)*
(iii) Intraduct papilloma
Ductal carcinoma *in situ* (DCIS)
Duct ectasia   *(3 marks)*

(b)   Cytology on nipple discharge
Mammography and/or ultrasonography
FNAC of a palpable lesion
Wire-guided excision biopsy   *(3 marks)*

Comment

Duct papilloma, common between the ages of 35 and 50 years, usually presents with a blood-stained nipple discharge as the only symptom. On examination a lump may be felt beneath the areola. Removal of the papilloma and the involved duct (microdochectomy) or ducts (major duct excision) is curative. However, a ductal carcinoma may have an identical clinical presentation and would necessitate a mastectomy after biopsy confirmation.

Answer 8

(a) (i) Size, consistency and mobility of lump
Attachment to overlying skin or chest wall
(2 marks)

(ii) Axillary nodes
Supraclavicular nodes
Internal mammary chain
Inferior epigastric chain *(2 marks)*

(b) Ultrasonography
Mammogram
FNAC or Image-guided core needle biopsy *(2 marks)*

(c) Removal of the entire breast or wide local excision, with axillary nodal sampling/clearance
Radiotherapy
Chemotherapy
Hormonal manipulation *(4 marks)*

Comment

Core needle biopsy, FNAC and ultrasonographic and mammographic findings are graded from benign to obviously malignant. Sentinel node biopsy of the axilla is performed following a positive diagnosis of breast cancer to determine axillary nodal status. A positive histological diagnosis is required before ablative surgery is performed. Counselling for breast reconstruction is necessary as reconstruction may be performed at the time of the mastectomy.

Answer 9

(a) (i) Infiltrating ductal (scirrhous)
carcinoma *(1 mark)*

(ii) Palpate right axilla and supraclavicular fossa
Examine contralateral breast and abdomen
Chest radiograph and bone scan
Liver scan and pelvic ultrasound
examination *(3 marks)*

(b) (i) Yes *(1 mark)*

(ii) Wide local excision, with hormone therapy
in hormone receptor positive tumours *(2 marks)*

(iii) The lesion may persist unchanged for a
considerable period of time before metastasising.
It is possible that she may die in the meantime of
an unrelated cause *(3 marks)*

Comment

Scirrhous tumours in elderly people are usually slow growing and
slow to metastasise. Surgical treatment should, therefore, be
confined to local removal. If surgery is declined, a course of
radiotherapy, with tamoxifen, may shrink the tumour and
improve the prognosis. There is little place for adjunct
chemotherapy. Approximately a half to a third of these tumours
are oestrogen or progesterone receptor positive and respond
favourably to tamoxifen, lefrazole or anastrezole.

Answer 10

(a) Mammography (or obtain screening mammograms)
Ultrasonography of breast
Image-guided FNAC or core needle biopsy *(3 marks)*

(b) Liver function tests, chest radiograph
Ultrasonography and/or isotope liver scan
Radionuclide bone scan

Bone marrow aspiration biopsy
Brain scan (only if indicated)   *(3 marks)*

(c)   Mastectomy or breast-conserving surgery with sentinel
      needle biopsy and if node positive axillary clearance
      Radiotherapy to the breast after wide local excision and
      to the axilla (instead of axillary surgery)
      Adjuvant chemotherapy for distant spread is
      based on tumour grade and nodal status   *(4 marks)*

Comment

Palpable and impalpable breast lesions may be graded by
mammography and ultrasonography as well as by cytology or core
needle biopsy to determine malignancy. If these findings are
equivocal, stereotactically guided wire localisation enables
impalpable lesions to be located and removed for histology.
Definitive cancer surgery should not be performed on the basis of
any one positive parameter, i.e. clinical, cytological or imaging
(positive cytology must be supported by ultrasonography and
mammography or core needle biopsy). Breast-conserving
operations remove small, unifocal cancers (< 4 cm in size).
Axillary node dissection assists in mainly for the staging of the
disease for adjuvant therapy.

7

ANSWERS

Cardiothoracic Surgery

Answer 1

(a) (i) Congenital diaphragmatic hernia *(1 mark)*

(ii) Mediastinal shift to the right
Presence of bowel and/or gastric gas
shadows in left pleural cavity
Collapse/compression of left lung *(3 marks)*

(b) Acute respiratory distress caused by gastric dilatation,
leading to collapse and consolidation of the affected
lung
Volvulus of herniated stomach
Acute bowel obstruction, which may lead to
perforation of herniated bowel loop *(3 marks)*

(c) Surgical reduction of abdominal contents from the
pleural cavity and excision of the herniated sac
Repair of defect in left diaphragm
Re-expansion of left lung
Ventilatory support in the postoperative
period *(3 marks)*

Comment
The usual sites of congenital diaphragmatic hernias are the foramen
of Bochdalek (pleuroperitoneal hernia), oesophageal hiatus,
foramen of Morgagni (anteriorly) and the dome. The condition
must be distinguished from acute respiratory distress syndrome,
oesophageal atresia and hypertrophic pyloric stenosis. Occasionally
the child may present with impending or actual obstruction of the
herniated bowel loop. Radiological features are, therefore, important
in establishing the diagnosis.

Answer 2

(a) An empyema thoracis is the diagnosis. Pre-operative work-up, including lung function studies
Single lung anaesthesia
Thoracotomy: decortication with evacuation of inflammatory tissue and pus   *(4 marks)*

(b) General anaesthesia: left lateral position with right arm supported on an armrest
Aseptic skin preparation
Insertion of fibreoptic scope into pleural space through a laterally placed stab incision in the second to fifth intercostal space
Structures visualised: lung surface, adhesions and fluid in pleural space
Pleural biopsies and fluid aspiration
Tissue samples sent for histology, and microbiological culture, including TB   *(3 marks)*

(c) Complication of chronic lung infections, e.g. lung abscess
Organisms: TB, *Staphylococcus aureus*
Iatrogenic introduction of infection into pleural space (during diagnostic needle aspiration)   *(3 marks)*

Comment

The thoracoscopy would have been preceded by chest radiograph and CT or MRI to localise the primary lesion in the lung. A primary tumour of the lung or pleura may give rise to these symptoms but a pyogenic or tubercular lung lesion is more common. In immunocompromised patients, chronic lung infections with atypical organisms frequently lead to pulmonary complications, such as abscess formation and empyema.

Answer 3

(a)   Papillary carcinoma of thyroid
Bronchial carcinoma
Breast carcinoma
Gastric carcinoma
Pancreatic carcinoma   *(2 marks)*

(b)   Bronchial small cell carcinoma
Chest radiograph (posteroanterior[PA], including lateral views)
Sputum for cytology
Bronchoscopy with brush and tissue biopsies for cytology and histology, respectively
Whole-body CT scan for metastases   *(4 marks)*

(c)   Removal of primary tumour (lobectomy or pneumonectomy) and regional lymph nodes
Adjuvant chemotherapy   *(4 marks)*

Comment

Small cell carcinomas account for 15% and squamous and adenocarcinomas for 70% of all lung cancers. Mediastinoscopy for nodal visualisation and biopsy indicates the extent of mediastinal nodal involvement by tumour. When contralateral nodes are involved surgery is contra-indicated. 20% of patients with lung cancer are considered suitable for surgery. Most patients receive palliation with chemotherapy.

Answer 4

(a)   Non-small cell lung cancer (NSCLC) accounts for approximately 75% of all lung cancers. NSCLC is divided further into:
- Adenocarcinoma (35–40%)
- Bronchoalveolar carcinoma (10–15%)
- Squamous cell carcinoma (25–30%)
- Large cell carcinoma (10–15%)   *(4 marks)*

(b) Apart from a handful of asymptomatic patients, in whom lung cancer is diagnosed incidentally, virtually all patients with lung cancer are symptomatic at presentation. In the presence of a long history of smoking or other risk factors for lung cancer, the presence of persistent respiratory symptoms should prompt a chest radiograph. Because benign conditions and metastatic malignancies can mimic lung cancer on radiographs, histologic confirmation is necessary. This can be achieved by sputum cytologic studies, bronchoscopy, or CT-guided transthoracic needle biopsy of the mass, depending on the location of the tumour. *(3 marks)*

(c) Surgical resection provides the best chance of long-term disease-free survival and possibility of a cure. Surgery in the form of lobectomy or pneumonectomy is the treatment of choice for stages I and II NSCLC. The role of surgery for stage III disease is controversial. Patients with completely resectable primary tumours (ie, T4 N0) have a much better prognosis than those with spread to ipsilateral mediastinal or subcarinal lymph nodes (ie, N2), signifying that spread beyond the primary tumour is associated with a poor prognosis. Patients with stage IIIB or IV tumours are generally not surgical candidates. *(3 marks)*

Answer 5

(a) Pleural mesothelioma *(1 mark)*

(b) Pleural mesothelioma usually begins as discrete plaques and nodules that coalesce to produce a sheetlike neoplasm. Tumour growth usually begins at the lower part of the chest. The tumour may invade the diaphragm and encase the surface of the lung and interlobar fissures.

The tumour may also grow along drainage and thoracotomy tracts. As the disease progresses, it often extends into the pulmonary parenchyma, chest wall, and mediastinum. Pleural mesothelioma may extend into the oesophagus, ribs, vertebra, brachial plexus, and superior vena cava.

Asbestos is the principal carcinogen implicated in the pathogenesis. *(3 marks)*

(c) Diagnosis of mesothelioma is made by performing thoracoscopically guided biopsy. Results are diagnostic in 98% of cases.

Careful scrutiny of routinely stained biopsy preparations is the most valuable diagnostic tool for making a diagnosis. *(3 marks)*

(d) Treatment options for the management of malignant mesothelioma include surgery, chemotherapy, radiation, and multimodality treatment.

Surgery in patients with disease confined to the pleural space is reasonable. Surgical resection has been relied upon because radiation and chemotherapy have been ineffective primary treatments. The surgical procedures used are pleurectomy with decortication and extrapleural pneumonectomy. These involve dissection of the parietal pleura; division of the pulmonary vessels; and *en bloc* resection of the lung, pleura, pericardium, and diaphragm followed by reconstruction. Surgery provides the best local control because it removes the entire pleural sac along with the lung parenchyma. *(3 marks)*

Answer 6

(a) Aortic sclerosis is the most common cause of aortic stenosis (AS) in elderly patients.

The most common cause of AS in patients < 70 years is a congenital bicuspid aortic valve.

In developing countries, rheumatic fever is the most common cause in all age groups. *(3 marks)*

(b)   The left ventricle (LV) gradually hypertrophies in response to AS. Significant LV hypertrophy causes diastolic dysfunction and, with progression, may lead to decreased contractility, ischaemia, or fibrosis, any of which may cause systolic dysfunction and heart failure (HF).   *(2 marks)*

(c)   For all practical purposes, there are two main options available for valve replacement. These are:
   •   Prosthetic valves created from synthetic material (mechanical prosthesis)
   •   Prosthetic valves fashioned from biological tissue (bioprosthesis).
   Three main designs of mechanical valves exist: the caged ball valve, the tilting disc (single leaflet) valve, and the bileaflet valve. Bioprosthetic (xenograft) valves are made from porcine valves or bovine pericardium. Homografts or preserved human aortic valves are used in a minority of patients.
   In some patients (usually young patients, athletes, women of child bearing age) pulmonary autograft can be used for aortic valve replacement. This procedure is termed Ross operation.   *(2 marks)*

(d) Traditionally, a mechanical valve has been used in patients < 65 years and in older patients with a long life expectancy, because bioprosthetic valves deteriorate over 10 to 12 years. Patients with a mechanical valve require lifelong anticoagulation to an international normalised ratio (INR) of 2.5 to 3.5 (to prevent thromboembolism) and antibiotics before some medical or dental procedures (to prevent endocarditis). A bioprosthetic valve, which does not require anticoagulation, has been used in patients > 65 years, younger patients with a life expectancy < 10 years, and those with some right-sided lesions. However, newer bioprosthetic valves may be more durable than 1st-generation valves; thus, patient preference regarding valve type can now be considered.   *(3 marks)*

Answer 7

(a) (i)   Ischaemic heart disease   *(1 mark)*

    (ii) ECG, echocardiogram   *(1 mark)*

    (iii) Ischaemic changes in pre-cordial leads
Myocardial and valvular functional defects

(2 marks)

(b) Coronary angiography defines the site(s), extent and degree of stenosis and treatment involves balloon angioplasty and/or insertion of coronary stents to revascularise diseased vessels   *(3 marks)*

(c) Coronary artery bypass grafting (CABG) of diseased vessels using the internal mammary or gastroepiploic artery, or long saphenous vein. The operation is performed by use of extracorporeal circulation, with systemic anticoagulation   *(3 marks)*

Comment

Balloon angioplasty and CABG have been shown to reduce myocardial infarcts significantly in patients with critical cardiac ischaemia. Bypass grafting is indicated when the angiogram shows extensive narrowing of two or more coronary vessels not amenable to angioplasty.

Answer 8

(a) The right and left coronary arteries arise from the right and left coronary sinuses in the root of the aorta just above the aortic valve orifice. The left coronary artery begins as the left main stem artery and quickly divides into the left anterior descending (LAD) and circumflex arteries. The left coronary artery mainly supplies the left ventricle. The right coronary artery supplies the sinus node (in 55% cases), right ventricle, and usually the AV node and inferior myocardial wall.   *(3 marks)*

(b) The conduits used for coronary artery bypass grafting can be broadly divided into two main types:
    (1) Arterial grafts (eg, left internal mammary artery, radial artery)
    (2) Venous grafts (eg, long or short saphenous vein)
Patency of arterial grafts is better than that of vein grafts.

(2 marks)

(c) Cardiopulmonary bypass (CPB) is a technique that temporarily takes over the function of the heart and lungs during surgery. It also maintains the circulation of blood and the oxygen content of the body. The CPB pump itself is often referred to as a Heart-Lung Machine. Cardiopulmonary bypass is commonly used in heart surgery because of the difficulty of operating on the beating heart. Operations requiring the opening of the chambers of the heart require the use of CPB to support the circulation during that period. *(2 marks)*

(d) Cardiopulmonary bypass provides the surgeon with a still field, absence of blood in the anastomotic area, and an empty flaccid heart that can be manipulated easily to expose all coronary branches. On the other hand, non-physiologic nature of the CPB leads to a propagation of the systemic inflammatory response with resultant complement and neutrophil activation, coagulopathy, alteration in fluid balance, renal, pulmonary and cardiovascular dysfunction, and stroke. *(3 marks)*

8

Upper Alimentary Tract

Answer 1

(a) Submandibular sialolithiasis (calculus) *(1 mark)*

(b) The simplest investigation to confirm the diagnosis is a conventional plain radiograph. AP, lateral and oblique intraoral occlusal views are used. This technique will diagnose the presence of radio-opaque calculi in about 70% of cases. However, these radiographs are limited in that they do not provide any information about the ductal system or soft tissues. *(2 marks)*

(c) Sjögren's disease, pleomorphic/monomorphic adenoma, chronic sialadenitis *(3 marks)*

(d) Salivary stagnation with epithelial injury along the salivary duct results in precipitation of calcium salts leading to sialolith formation. This sialolith acts as a nidus for further stone formation. *(2 marks)*

(e) Salivary calculi are managed as follows:
- Medical management: hydration, compression and massage, antibiotics for the infected gland
- Surgical management: duct cannulation with stone removal, and gland excision in recurrent cases

(2 marks)

Answer 2

(a) (i) Pleomorphic adenoma of parotid gland   *(1 mark)*
    (ii) Size and location
         Per oral examination of fauces for involvement of
         deep part of gland
         Involvement of branches of the facial nerve
         (3 marks)

(b) Contraindicated as a result of seeding of tumour
    along the needle track to skin   *(2 marks)*

(c) (i) A conservative superficial parotidectomy
        (conservative total parotidectomy with
        preservation of the facial nerve branches if the
        deep part of the gland is involved)   *(3 marks)*
    (ii) Facial nerve trunk and its five branches must be
         preserved   *(1 mark)*

Comment

Pleomorphic adenomas are locally invasive and 'shelling out' the
tumour invariably leads to recurrence; re-exploration may
compromise the facial nerve and its branches. Dissection of the
facial nerve branches during removal of the deep portion of the
gland leads to transient facial palsy in the post-operative period
and is a result of neuropraxia from bruising or tissue swelling.

Answer 3

(a) (i) Ludwig's angina (acute cellulitis of the
        submandibular and cervical regions)
        Inflammation and swelling of tissue planes
        superficial and deep to the investing layer of the
        deep cervical fascia, involving the
        submandibular region   *(2 marks)*
    (ii) *Streptococcus* spp.
         Vincent's organisms
         Gram-negative anaerobes   *(2 marks)*

(b) (i) The inflammatory oedema extends deep to the investing layer of the deep cervical fascia at and above the level of the hyoid bone, involving the glottis and displacing the tongue upwards and out through the mouth, leading to the imminent danger of asphyxiation   *(2 marks)*

(ii) Rehydration and analgesia

Intravenous amoxicillin or a cephalosporin with metronidazole gives broad-spectrum therapy and usually leads to rapid resolution

If resolution is delayed, surgical decompression and drainage of the submandibular space under local infiltration anaesthesia are required   *(4 marks)*

Comment

Ludwig's angina is an infection of a closed fascial space and, if untreated, the inflammatory exudate may track along the stylohyoid muscle to the submucosa of the glottis, when the patient is in danger of asphyxiation from glottic oedema.

Surgical decompression is through a curved incision beneath the mandible, displacing the submandibular gland and dividing the mylohyoid muscles, thereby opening up the fascial space.

Answer 4

(a) An ulcer with slough on an indurated base and everted edges

Pain

Salivation

Ankyloglossia

Dysphagia

Inability to articulate clearly

Alteration in the voice

Fetor oris

Lump in the neck as a result of cervical nodal spread   *(3 marks)*

(b) Leukoplakia
Smoking
Spirits (alcohol)
Spices
Sepsis
Friction (from sharp edge of tooth)
Syphilis
Candidiasis   *(3 marks)*

(c) *In situ* and small (< 1 cm) tumours are excised with a
1 cm clear margin. Lesions < 2 cm are treated by
interstitial irradiation using caesium needles or iridium
wire

For lesions > 2 cm external beam irradiation is used.
Tumours with cervical nodal metastases are treated
with a combination of radiotherapy and block
dissection of the neck nodes   *(4 marks)*

Comment

Leukoplakia is regarded as a pre-cancerous condition. When
causative irritants are identified and avoided, early lesions resolve.
Surgical excision of cancerous lesions on the tongue is limited
because of the resulting functional disability. Except for the very
small lesions, all tongue cancers are treated with radiotherapy. The
place of chemotherapy is undecided.

Answer 5

(a) (i) Oesophageal atresia with/without tracheo-
oesophageal fistula   *(1 mark)*
(ii) Gastrograffin swallow   *(1 mark)*

(b) (i) 85% incidence – most common form   *(4 marks)*

(Trachea and bronchi are shaded)

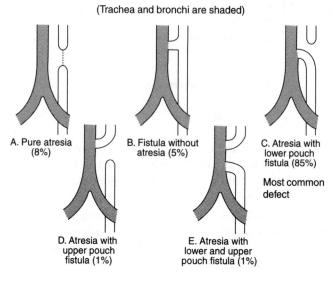

A. Pure atresia (8%)

B. Fistula without atresia (5%)

C. Atresia with lower pouch fistula (85%)

Most common defect

D. Atresia with upper pouch fistula (1%)

E. Atresia with lower and upper pouch fistula (1%)

   (ii)   Passage of nasal feeding tube into stomach to confirm oesophageal patency by aspirating stomach contents   *(2 marks)*

(c)   Transthoracic excision of oesophageal atresia and associated tracheo-oesophageal fistula, with restoration of oesophageal continuity and repair of tracheal defect   *(2 marks)*

Comment

Oesophageal atresia must be diagnosed at birth to prevent the aspiration pneumonitis that rapidly ensues. The simple procedure of passing a nasal feeding catheter at birth and testing the aspirate with litmus would exclude all oesophagea anomalies except tracheo-oesophageal fistula without oesophageal atresia (Type B).

Answer 6

   (a)   Achalasia   *(1 mark)*

   (b)   Achalasia is characterised by the following clinical features:
- Dysphagia (most common)
- Regurgitation

- Chest pain
- Heart burn
- Weight loss
- Physical examination is non-contributory

(3 marks)

(c) The investigations performed to aid the diagnosis include:
- Barium swallow or OGD
- Oesophageal manometry
- Prolonged oesophageal pH monitoring

(3 marks)

(d) Achalasia is managed as follows:
- Medical management: calcium channel blockers and nitrates or intrasphincteric injection of botulinum toxin for elderly patients with contraindications for pneumatic dilatation or surgery.
- Pneumatic dilatation: performed by a gastroenterologist when surgery is not appropriate.
- Surgical management: laparoscopic or open Heller myotomy. *(3 marks)*

Answer 7

(a) Dysphagia for solids and/or liquids
Pain on swallowing
Retrosternal pain/discomfort
Vomiting old food
Aspiration of saliva, leading to recurrent chest infections
Site of obstruction as felt by patient *(2 marks)*

(b) (i) Bulbar (and pseudobulbar) palsy
Extra-oesophageal compression caused by mediastinal tumours
Iron-deficiency anaemia
Pharyngeal pouch
Oesophageal causes:
  scleroderma

                inflammatory stricture
                malignant stricture
                achalasia   *(3 marks)*

    (ii)   Barium swallow: outlines the lesion and
           defines the anatomical site
           Oesophagogastroduodenoscopy (OGD):
           visualisation and biopsy of lesion   *(2 marks)*

(c)   Aetiology: hiatus hernia produces reflux oesophagitis
      and stricture
      Malignant stricture: smoking and alcohol or Barrett's
      oesophagus produces squamous metaplasia and
      may lead to anaplasia   *(3 marks)*

Comment

The oesophagus is inaccessible to clinical examination; consequently, a working diagnosis of oesophageal cancer must be based on the presenting symptoms and confirmed by endoscopy or imaging. Occasionally a patient may present with respiratory symptoms caused by aspiration or tumour extension into the trachea or bronchus. Surgery is aimed at removing the tumour and restoring continuity by bringing the stomach up into the chest or by interposing a loop of large bowel. Radiotherapy is a viable treatment option, because squamous carcinomas are radiosensitive.

Adenocarcinomas of the gastric fundus may extend into the oesophagus, producing dysphagia. Surgery entails an oesophagoproximal gastrectomy and restoring continuity, using either the distal gastric remnant or a jejunal roux loop.

Answer 8

    (a) (i)   Hiatus hernia   *(1 mark)*
         (ii)   Herniation of portion of stomach into left
             pleural cavity, leading to a sliding or rolling
             hernia, which results in oesophageal ulceration
             and bleeding, and later oesophageal stricture in
             the former. Squamous metaplasia may occur in
             the portion of the stomach that slides into the
             chest, giving rise to Barrett's oesophagus, a
             premalignant condition   *(3 marks)*

    (iii) Barium swallow or OGD *(1 mark)*

(b) (i) Erect and semi-recumbent posture at work and sleep
Antireflux medication (alginate preparations, antacids)
Reduce gastric acid production with H_2-receptor blockade or proton pump inhibition
Weight reduction *(2 marks)*
(ii) An antireflux operation, such as the Nissen fundoplication or the Leigh–Collis gastroplasty performed through the abdomen, or the Belsey repair performed through the chest *(3 marks)*

Comment

Treatment of hiatus hernia is aimed at relief of symptoms. A dramatic improvement occurs after weight reduction in those who are overweight. Many operations have been devised because none has been entirely satisfactory. The Nissen fundoplication is probably the procedure used most often and is now performed laparoscopically.

Answer 9

(a) (i) Hypertrophic pyloric stenosis *(2 marks)*
(ii) Achalasia of the cardia
Duodenal atresia
Annular pancreas *(2 marks)*
(iii) The hypertrophied pylorus ('pyloric tumour') *(1 mark)*

(b) Hypertrophy of the circular smooth muscle fibres of the pylorus producing a functional gastric outlet obstruction *(2 marks)*

(c) Medical measures: rehydration; smooth muscle relaxants (e.g. hyoscine) before feeds
Surgery: division of all hypertrophied muscle fibres without breaching the mucosa *(3 marks)*

Comment

The palpation of an enlarged pylorus after a feed, with the infant preferably asleep, is diagnostic of hypertrophic stenosis and imaging is unnecessary. Medical measures are not generally successful.

Answer 10

(a) (i) Peptic ulcer disease   *(1 mark)*

    (ii) Stressful lifestyle
          Helicobacter pylori infection
          Alcohol and smoking
          Irregular meals   *(2 marks)*

(b) OGD
       Sedation (midazolam 2–5 mg i.v.)
       Mouth guard and anaesthetic throat spray
       Visualisation through endoscope or on video screen
       Endoscopic biopsy via biopsy channel   *(2 marks)*

(c) (i) Adopt healthy lifestyle measures
          Stop oral intake of anti-inflammatory agents
          Eradication of *H. pylori* by broad-spectrum antibiotics (amoxicillin and clarithromycin or metronidazole), with H_2-receptor blockade (cimetidine, ranitidine) or proton pump inhibition (omeprazole or lansoprazole)
          Surgery (anti-acid procedure) for failed medical therapy and complications   *(3 marks)*

    (ii) Complications of peptic ulceration: bleeding, perforation, stenosis causing gastric outlet obstruction
          Chronic prepyloric ulceration may predispose to gastric carcinoma   *(2 marks)*

Comment

The importance of stress, alcohol and tobacco in the aetiology of this disease requires the implementation of 'lifestyle measures' aimed at reducing these factors and promoting health.

Since the advent of effective medical measures in ulcer healing, surgery for peptic ulcer disease is reserved for the complications of bleeding, perforation, stenosis and possible malignancy.

An antiulcer procedure involves denervation of the stomach (vagotomy) and drainage of the denervated stomach (by a pyloroplasty or gastroenterostomy) or removal of the acid-secreting portion of the stomach.

Answer 11

(a) Test for the presence of urease (Heli's test) for evidence of *Helicobacter pylori*
Haematoxylin and eosin stain for evidence of type II gastritis and/or the presence of *H. pylori*
Culture isolation *(3 marks)*

(b) (i) *H. pylori* *(1 mark)*
(ii) Treatment regimens involve gastric acid suppression and antibiotic therapy; these include clarithromycin 500 mg twice daily, either omeprazole 20 mg or lansoprazole 500 mg twice daily and either metronidazole 400 mg or tinidazole 500 mg twice daily *(3 marks)*

(c) *H. pylori* is found in type II gastritis. It raises the local pH by ammonia production and may thereby cause mucosal damage, leading to ulceration. The persistence of infection leads to chronicity and gastric ulcers may predispose to malignancy *(3 marks)*

Comment

H. pylori infection has been implicated in the aetiology of peptic ulcer disease. H_2-receptor blockers or proton pump inhibitors reduce gastric acid production, but to achieve permanent ulcer healing requires eradication of the underlying *H. pylori* infection and the chronic gastritis that it produces.

Answer 12

(a) (i) Peritonitis caused by peptic ulcer
perforation *(2 marks)*

    (ii) Free gas on erect abdominal radiograph, i.e.
under right diaphragm and between bowel loops
Inflammatory thickening of the pre-peritoneal
fat layer in the abdominal wall *(2 marks)*

(b) Intravenous analgesia and antibiotics
Intravenous fluids; nasogastric aspiration
Consent for emergency laparotomy
Closure of perforation and peritoneal toilet with
definitive anti-ulcer surgery in selected patients

(4 marks)

(c) Stop or change anti-inflammatory agent to one that is
less ulcerogenic
Commence long term anti-ulcer
medication *(2 marks)*

Comment

Emergency surgery is mandatory in a perforated viscus due to
lethal complications of peritonitis. In a young and otherwise fit
patient with a peptic perforation, recurrent ulceration may be
prevented by an anti-ulcer operation during the emergency
surgery. Very occasionally a 'pin-hole' perforation with limited
peritoneal contamination may be non-surgically managed in the
expectation that the perforation would seal itself; close monitoring
with IV omeprazole therapy is essential to assess response.

Answer 13

(a) Troisier's sign: nodal metastases at the root of the neck,
usually from a gastric carcinoma
FNAC or biopsy of the node may reveal an
adenocarcinoma originating from the upper GI tract

(2 marks)

(b) Gastroscopy and mucosal biopsy
Double-contrast barium meal
CT or MRI   *(3 marks)*

(c) Macroscopically recognised types are:
Type 1: cauliflower-like lesion
Type 2: ulcer–cancer
Type 3: colloid carcinoma
Type 4: scirrhous carcinoma (linitis plastica)
Type 5: carcinoma in a previously benign gastric ulcer
Definitive treatment:
> Localised lesions (types 1, 2 and 5): partial or
> subtotal gastrectomy
> Diffuse lesions (types 3 and 4): total gastrectomy

Palliative treatment:
> Unresectable lesions – surgical bypass or
> endoscopic intubation to facilitate gastric
> emptying chemotherapy   *(5 marks)*

Comment

Gastric cancers usually present insidiously or with a diversity of symptoms; there appears to be a considerable time lapse between the appearance of the cancer and its clinical manifestations. Pancreatic tumours also have a similar presentation. Laparoscopy assesses the feasibility of resection. Radical surgery for the early lesion, which includes removal of the regional lymph nodes, offers the best hope of a cure. The presentation of an epigastric mass lesion with/without jaundice indicates an advanced lesion, with impending gastric outlet or biliary obstruction. Bypass surgery with chemotherapy offers the best palliation.

Answer 14

(a) Immediate control of bleeding by
Sengstaken–Blakemore tube placement or endoscopic sclerotherapy or banding and intravenous vasopressin
If these measures fail, consider oesophageal
transection or emergency portasystemic
shunt   *(4 marks)*

(b) Chronic liver damage (e.g. hepatitis B infection or alcohol abuse) predisposes to cirrhosis, which in turn leads to portal hypertension and variceal bleeding *(3 marks)*

(c) Follow up every 3–6 months with oesophagoscopy and prophylactic sclerotherapy or banding of recurrent varices. Long term follow up is mandatory *(3 marks)*

Comment

Treatment of gastro-oesophageal varices is palliative unless the underlying portal hypertension is curable. Elective surgical shunts (splenorenal, mesocaval and portacaval) require satisfactory liver function (Child's groups A and B) to be effective. In selected cases orthopic liver transplantation has been successful.

Answer 15

(a) Primary haemorrhage: during surgery, from uncontrolled bleeding points
Reactionary haemorrhage after return to normal BP
Secondary haemorrhage occurs a few days later, as a result of infection *(3 marks)*

(b) Quarter-hourly BP, pulse and respiratory rate, and CVP monitoring
Examination of abdominal wound and abdominal girth measurement
Resuscitation if required
Blood volume replacement
Emergency surgical re-exploration and haemostasis *(4 marks)*

(c) Pneumococcal infection caused by fall in cell-mediated immunity
Prophylaxis: pneumovaccine
Antibiotic (phenoxymethylpenicillin) cover for future invasive procedures *(3 marks)*

Comment

Postoperative bleeding from uncontrolled bleeding points into body cavities, such as the chest and abdomen, may go unnoticed until the patient lapses into oligaemic shock. Suitably placed drains assist in its early detection, and close monitoring of vital signs enables timely resuscitation and surgical control.

To preserve immunological functions of the spleen, a small portion of the spleen may be re-implanted during splenectomy for splenic trauma. In children, the spleen should be salvaged if possible by repairing the laceration.

9

ANSWERS

Liver, Gallbladder and Pancreas

Answer 1

(a) Infective:
   Malaria
   Schistosomiasis
   Hydatid disease
   Kala-azar
Blood dyscrasias:
   Chronic leukaemia
   Polycythaemia rubra vera
   Sickle cell disease
   Thalassaemia
   Hereditary spherocytosis
Circulatory:
   Portal hypertension
Autoimmune disease:
   Felty's syndrome
   Still's syndrome
Neoplastic:
   Hodgkin's and non-Hodgkin's lymphomas *(3 marks)*

(b) Hypersplenism is splenic enlargement with the sequestration and/or destruction of peripheral blood cells in the splenic circulation; this results in anaemia, leukopenia and/or thrombocytopenia *(3 marks)*

(c) A grossly enlarged spleen is at increased risk of rupture, either spontaneously or after mild trauma; the medical indications are:

Hypersplenism
Hereditary spherocytosis
Idiopathic thrombocytopenic purpura
Autoimmune haemolytic anaemias
Felty's syndrome
Tropical splenomegaly syndrome
Hydatid disease
Schistosomiasis
Staging of Hodgkin's disease
Primary splenic tumours
Pyruvate kinase deficiency   *(4 marks)*

Comment

A grossly enlarged spleen is invariably associated with hypersplenism and is also prone to rupture from blunt trauma. Elective splenectomy is indicated for the correction of specific haematological abnormalities, in the treatment of some blood cancers and in the staging of Hodgkin's disease.

Answer 2

(a) (i) Calculus cholecystitis   *(1 mark)*
   (ii) Murphy's sign
      Palpable gallbladder
      Paraesthesiae over the right upper quadrant
      and back   *(2 marks)*
   (iii) Ultrasonography of the gallbladder and
       biliary tree   *(1 mark)*

(b) Increasing concentrations of cholesterol, bile pigments and lecithin in the bile, with a reduction in the bile acid pool, leads to cholesterol, pigment and calcium salt supersaturation. In the absence of glycoprotein crystallisation inhibitors and impaired gallbladder motility and/or infection, these compounds crystallise to form stones   *(3 marks)*

(c) Remove inflamed gallbladder by open or laparoscopic cholecystectomy. During the procedure image for stones in the biliary tree by peroperative cholangiogram and explore the bile duct to remove duct stones indicated   *(3 marks)*

Comment

The classic symptoms of cholecystitis that follow a fatty meal are the result of cholecystokinin secreted by the presence of fat in the duodenum, which stimulates a diseased gallbladder to contract, usually against a stone. Nonfunctioning gallbladders, despite containing stones, may remain silent for this reason. There is, therefore, no indication for treating asymptomatic gallstones.

Answer 3

(a) (i) Ascending cholangitis   *(1 mark)*
   (ii) Migration of gallstones from gallbladder into bile duct → obstruction → biliary stasis → ascending infection   *(2 marks)*
   (iii) Hb and WBC to detect anaemia and sepsis
   LFTs to indicate extent of liver damage by obstruction to bile flow and sepsis
   Serum amylase, if elevated, suggests pancreatic duct obstruction, with pancreatitis
   Blood cultures: aerobic and anaerobic may isolate offending organism(s)   *(3 marks)*

(b) Ultrasonography and imidoacetic acid excretion (HIDA) scans of the liver and biliary tree   *(1 mark)*

(c) Rehydration with intravenous fluids
   Analgesia
   Correct anaemia
   Treat infection with intravenous antibiotics
   Drain biliary tree by percutaneous transhepatic catheter, ERCP and endoscopic sphincterotomy, or surgical drainage of bile duct, with cholecystectomy   *(3 marks)*

Comment

Cholangiohepatitis in western societies is caused by ascending infection as a result of migrating gallstones or rarely primary hepatic stones obstructing the common bile duct. It is important to distinguish this from viral hepatitis, which is largely a self-limiting illness. As progressive liver damage occurs, the biliary tree must be decompressed as an emergency, by means of a transhepatic catheter. Planned surgical or endoscopic drainage should follow.

Answer 4

(a) (i) Accidental injury or ligation of the
common hepatic or bile duct *(1 mark)*

(ii) Percutaneous transhepatic cholangiogram *— to view biliary tree*
(PTC) *(1 mark)*

(iii) Chest radiograph, coagulation screen
Vitamin K prophylaxis
Blood group and crossmatch *(2 marks)*

(b) Bile leak causing peritonitis as a result of partial/complete division of the bile duct or ischaemic injury to the liver from right hepatic arterial occlusion *(2 marks)*

(c) Good exposure and visualisation of the surgical field
Identification of anatomy of Callot's triangle
Per-operative cholangiogram
Immediate T-tube drainage after accidental injury to the bile duct *(4 marks)*

Comment

Damage to the hepatic or bile ducts or right hepatic artery during cholecystectomy is an avoidable catastrophe. Technical inexpertise, along with the occasionally encountered anomalies of the hepatic artery and ducts, accounts for most of these misadventures. During laparoscopic cholecystectomy the surgeon should, on encountering technical difficulty, convert to an open operation. Peroperative cholangiogram assists in outlining the anatomy in a difficult dissection.

Answer 5

(a) (i)   Gallstone ileus *(1 mark)*

   (ii) Chronic calculus cholecystitis leading to erosion of the gallstone into the duodenum and its passage down the small bowel, with obstruction usually in the distal ileum *(1 mark)*

   (iii) Distended loops of small bowel
   Possible radio-opaque calculus in terminal ileum
   Air in the biliary tree *(2 marks)*

(b) Nasogastric aspiration
   Fluid and electrolyte replacement
   Adequate analgesia
   Emergency laparotomy and relief of obstruction with cholecystecomy *(3 marks)*

(c) Ultrasonography of gallbladder and biliary tree to confirm calculus disease and assess calibre of bile duct
   ERCP and sphincterotomy if duct stones are present *(3 marks)*

Comment

Gallstone ileus is an uncommon complication of cholelithiasis and, as a history of biliary disease may not be obvious (a proportion of gallstones being silent), air in the biliary tree on abdominal radiograph usually clarifies the diagnosis. The obstruction must be relieved surgically. The gallbladder may be found to be firmly adherent to the duodenum and should be removed and a duodenal fistula closed.

Answer 6

(a) (i)   Acute pancreatitis   *(1 mark)*
    (ii)   Biliary calculi
          Alcohol abuse   *(2 marks)*

(b) Resuscitate:
    Oxygen by facemask or nasal catheter
    Intravenous fluids
    Pain relief
    Nasogastric aspiration
    Intravenous broad-spectrum antibiotics
Monitor:
    Lung function and tissue oxygenation: respiratory rate and ABG estimation
    Circulation: BP, pulse rate and CVP measurement
    Liver and kidney function: U&Es, LFTs and urine output
    Pancreatic function: blood glucose and serum and urinary calcium estimations   *(4 marks)*

(c) Hypovolaemic shock
Respiratory failure
Renal failure
Secondary infection
Pseudocyst formation
Hypocalcaemia   *(3 marks)*

Comment

The course of acute pancreatitis is unpredictable, irrespective of the underlying cause. In a small minority of patients the disease is rapidly progressive, and early identification of this group enables close monitoring and support of cardiorespiratory and renal functions in an intensive care setting. Surgical intervention is restricted to complications of pancreatic haemorrhage or necrosis in fulminant disease, or of abscess or pseudocyst formation in subacute disease.

Answer 7

(a) Periampullary carcinoma or bile duct carcinoma
     Pancreatic, biliary and liver imaging by
     ultrasonography and CT
     ERCP
     Cytology on pancreatic juice and bile obtained at ERCP
     Percutaneous image-guided core needle biopsy
                                                          (3 marks)

(b) (i)   Supportive and hospice care
           Palliation by endoscopic or transhepatic stenting
           of malignant stricture
           Surgical palliation by biliary bypass operation
           Curative surgery: pancreatoduodenectomy
           (Whipple's operation)   *(3 marks)*
     (ii) Poor anaesthetic or surgical risk
           Advanced primary tumour
           Local and/or regional spread of tumour *(2 marks)*

(c) Haemorrhage
     Wound infection
     Wound dehiscence
     Delayed wound healing
     Renal failure   *(2 marks)*

Comment

Most ampullary and biliary tumours are beyond curative measures
on presentation and are treated palliatively. Pain is controlled by
opiates when required. Pancreatic supplements will aid digestion
and reduce weight loss. Pruritus is associated with jaundice and
both are relieved by stenting or bypassing the obstruction.

Answer 8

(a) (i)   Stress ulcer (Curling's ulcer) of the stomach or
              duodenum
              Haemobilia   *(1 mark)*
       (ii) Stress ulcer is treated by H$_2$-receptor or calcium
              blockade or proton pump inhibition
              Ulcer bleeding uncontrolled by the above
              measures may be treated by submucous injection
              of adrenaline or laser photocoagulation
              Haemobilia is the result of a traumatic fistula
              between a hepatic vessel and a branch of the
              biliary tree. It usually resolves, otherwise
              angiographic embolisation of the fistula is
              required   *(4 marks)*

(b) (i)   A pancreatic fistula   *(1 mark)*
       (ii) A fistulogram through the drainage tube or
              ERCP   *(2 marks)*
(c) (i)   A leak from damage to the bile duct
              system   *(1 mark)*
       (ii) An imidoacetic acid excretion (HIDA) scan or
              ERCP   *(1 mark)*

Comment

Complications of trauma to the bile duct or pancreas may present
late and represent unrecognised injury. Traumatic pancreatic
fistulae close on supportive measures alone if continuity of the
pancreatic duct is preserved. Complete transection, however,
rarely heals without surgical intervention. Pseudocyst formation is
a late complication of pancreatic injury. It resolves either
spontaneously or after ultrasound-guided aspirations, provided
that there is no underlying pancreatic disease.

Answer 9

(a) (i) A clinical label when an underlying causative
          factor has not been found   *(1 mark)*
     (ii) Obsessive–compulsive neuroses
          Attention-seeking behaviour patterns
          Anorexia nervosa and bulimic
          disorders   *(2 marks)*

(b) (i) Chronic relapsing pancreatitis
          A raised serum amylase
          A normal or low serum calcium
          Abdominal radiograph may show pancreatic
          calcification
          Abdominal ultrasonography may show
          pancreatic calculi, fibrosis or oedema   *(3 marks)*
     (ii) Abstinence from alcohol and a low-fat diet with
          pancreatic enzyme supplementation. When pain
          persists, despite patient compliance, it is usually a
          result of fibrosis of the duct; relief may be
          achieved by splanchnic nerve block

          Long-term pain relief using opiate analgesics may
          lead to habituation and drug dependency

          Surgical measures are restricted to complications
          such as chronic relapsing pancreatitis and
          intractable pain non-responsive to other
          measures   *(4 marks)*

Comment

Surgery is based on pancreatographic and CT findings. If the head
of the pancreas is diseased, a pancreatoduodenectomy is performed,
with the distal segment draining into the stomach or jejunum.
Involvement of the distal segment would require a distal
pancreatectomy. Occasionally the duct is grossly dilated as a result
of multiple stenoses; it is opened along its length by filleting the
gland, and drained into a loop of bowel (longitudinal
pancreatojejunostomy – Peustow's operation).

Small and Large Bowel

Answer 1

(a) (i) Exomphalos (omphalocele) *(1 mark)*

(ii) During intrauterine life a portion of the intestine lies outside the abdomen (between weeks 6 and 12)

As a result of an error in development, the intestine fails to return to the abdomen at birth, with a resultant defect in the abdominal wall *(3 marks)*

(b) Immediate surgery aimed at reducing the contents of the sac and closing the defect in the abdomen

The sac is covered with moist dressing to prevent rupture before surgery

If closure of the abdominal defect is not possible, a Silastic sheath may be sutured on to the abdominal wall until elective repair a few weeks later *(3 marks)*

(c) Oesophageal atresia (with or without tracheo-oesophageal fistula)
Duodenal atresia (also intestinal atresia)
Imperforate anus (anorectal malformation) *(3 marks)*

Comment

Exomphalos is when a portion of the alimentary tract lies outside the abdominal cavity enclosed by the umbilical cord. It differs from gastroschisis, where the abdominal contents are exteriorised through a defect in the abdominal wall adjacent to the umbilical cord.

When these anomalies are associated with a large defect or a poorly developed abdominal wall, it is inadvisable to attempt to reduce the contents and close the defect, because of ensuing respiratory complications. It may be possible to achieve skin cover alone, or a Silastic sheath may be sutured onto the opening and the contents gradually reduced by twisting the sheath over a period of time as the abdominal wall expands.

Answer 2

(a) Necrotising enterocolitis (NEC)   *(1 mark)*

(b) The aetiology of NEC is controversial, but is in all likelihood multifactorial. It is usually seen in preterm infants after oral feeding is instituted. Bacteria, ischaemic insult and platelet-activating factor contribute to increasing gut mucosal permeability and barrier breakdown.   *(3 marks)*

(c) The mainstay of diagnostic imaging is abdominal radiography. An anteroposterior (AP) abdominal radiograph and a left lateral decubitus radiograph (left side down) are essential for initially evaluating any baby with abdominal signs.   *(1 mark)*

(d) Characteristic findings on an AP abdominal radiograph include:
   •   an abnormal gas pattern
   •   dilated loops
   •   thickened bowel walls (suggesting oedema/inflammation}
   •   scarce or absent intestinal gas
   •   pneumatosis intestinalis
   •   abdominal free air indication bowel perforation
        (2 marks)

(e) Treatment of NEC depends on the degree of bowel involvement and severity of its presentation. Objective staging criteria developed by Bell have been widely adopted or modified to help tailor therapy according to disease severity.
Bell Stage I (Suspected disease)
- Stage IA & IB - NPO with antibiotics for 3 days.
Bell Stage II (Definite disease)
- Stage IIA (patient is mildly ill) - NPO and antibiotics for 7-10 days.
- Stage IIB (patient is moderately ill) - NPO and antibiotics for 14 days.

Bell stage III (Advanced NEC with severe illness that has a high likelihood of progressing to surgical intervention)
- Stage IIIA (patient has severe NEC with an intact bowel) - NPO for 14 days, fluid resuscitation, inotropic support, ventilator support, and paracentesis of abdomen.
- Stage IIIB (severely ill infant with perforated bowel observed on radiograph) - Free air visible on abdominal radiograph indicates surgery. Surgical treatment includes resecting the affected portion of the bowel, which may be extensive. Initially, an ileostomy with a mucous fistula is typically performed, with reanastomosis performed later.

(3 marks)

Answer 3

(a) Infective diarrhoea
Inflammatory bowel disease
Neoplasms, i.e. benign polyps, adenocarcinoma
or lymphoma   *(3 marks)*

(b) Sigmoidoscopy (rigid or flexible), followed by barium enema or colonoscopy, with full bowel preparation
Endoscopic mucosal biopsies   *(4 marks)*

(c) Ascitic tap for protein content and cytology

A low protein content would exclude an inflammatory cause, and the presence of neoplastic cells would suggest a disseminated colonic cancer

Liver ultrasonography or radio-isotope scan may reveal discrete lesions, such as a liver abscess or metastatic tumour deposits *(3 marks)*

Comment

Inflammatory bowel disease and bowel cancer have similar presentations. The former is incurable but treatable and compatible with a normal life expectancy. The latter has a favourable prognosis if detected early and a poor outcome when diagnosis is delayed. Ulcerative colitis carries a small but significant risk of colonic cancer over time. These patients must, therefore, be on colonoscopic surveillance.

Answer 4

(a) Pneumatosis intestinalis *(1 mark)*

(b) Bowel necrosis, immunosuppression, and severe obstructive pulmonary disease *(3 marks)*

(c) Pneumatosis intestinalis is a radiographic finding and not a diagnosis, as the aetiology varies from benign conditions to fulminant gastrointestinal disease. Pneumatosis intestinalis is considered an ominous finding in bowel ischaemia, particularly if it is associated with portomesenteric venous gas. *(2 marks)*

(d) Multiple factors can contribute to the development of pneumatosis intestinalis. Finding the underlying cause can help in tailoring the appropriate medical and/or surgical treatment of the patient. Most patients with primary pneumatosis intestinalis require no treatment.

Surgical intervention is recommended if the bowel
ischaemia or perforation is present. Surgery should be
performed in patients who are not responding to
nonoperative treatment, especially those with signs of
perforation, peritonitis, or abdominal sepsis. As many
as 50% of patients may require surgery for perforation.

(3 marks)

(e) In patients with pneumatosis intestinalis, the prognosis
depends on the overall clinical picture. The prognosis is
excellent in primary pneumatosis intestinalis (15% of
cases) while it is worse in cases where pneumatosis is
associated with obstructive and necrotic
gastrointestinal disease. *(1 mark)*

Answer 5

(a) (i) Acute bowel obstruction as a result of
intussusception *(1 mark)*
(ii) Aetiology:
Lymphoid hyperplasia in bowel wall as a
result of weaning and enteric viral infections
Childhood leukaemias and bowel
lymphomas *(2 marks)*

(b) Abdominal examination:
Distension, tympanitic, increased bowel sounds
Palpable mass
Per rectum: empty ampulla, possibly a pelvic
mass; 'redcurrant jelly' motions *(3 marks)*

(c) (i) Barium or gastrograffin enema *(1 mark)*
(ii) Under a light general anaesthetic dilute barium is
trickled into the rectum under a hydrostatic
pressure not exceeding 30 cmH$_2$O
Screening identifies the position and features of
the intussusception. The pressure is maintained
for a period (not exceeding 30 min) before re-
screening to assess reduction of the
intussusception *(3 marks)*

Comment

The presence of a mobile abdominal mass with 'redcurrant jelly' stool is diagnostic of an intussusception. Diluted barium or gastrograffin reduces the intussusception by hydrostatic pressure and thereby avoids an operation. However, when the diagnosis is delayed or the presentation late, even surgical reduction may prove difficult, because of the extensive oedema of the trapped bowel. Further, as the intussusception progresses, the blood supply is compromised, with infarction of the intussuscepted bowel loop.

Answer 6

(a) Dilated loops of jejunum and/or ileum with air–fluid levels
Absence of gas in bowel distal to obstruction　*(2 marks)*

(b) (i) Assessment of dehydration and electrolyte depletion: tongue moisture and skin turgor
U&Es and ABG estimation for electrolyte and acid–base balance
Monitor nasogastric aspirate (about 1000–2000 ml/24 h)
Urine output (about 1300 ml/24 h) and urine osmolarity
Insensible to fluid loss (about 700 ml/24 h)
　　　　　　　　　　　　　　　　　(3 marks)

(ii) Treat deficit and daily requirements by giving isotonic (0.9%) saline alternating with 5% dextrose or with one-fifth isotonic (0.18%) saline and 4.3% dextrose solution with an additional 60–100 mmol K^+ per 24 h (the dextrose provides 400–500 cal/24 h) Twice-daily haematocrit and U&E estimation and urine output guide the daily replacement　*(3 marks)*

(c) Drip-and-suck regimen
Keep patient in fluid and electrolyte balance
Failure to respond to the above measures may require laparotomy and division of adhesions　*(2 marks)*

Comment

The average adult requires 2000–3000 ml water containing at least 100 mmol Na^+ and 60 mmol K^+ daily. These requirements are increased by the degree of dehydration. However, great care must be exercised not to over-transfuse because 'to overload the circulation is a grievous fault, and grievously does the patient pay for it'. If normal bowel function does not return in a few days, parenteral alimentation (intravenous feeding) must be considered to prevent the breakdown of body proteins.

Answer 7

(a) Hirschsprung's disease
Anorectal malformations (i.e. rectal atresia, rectal stenosis, imperforate anus)   *(2 marks)*

(b) (i) Meconium ileus, Hirschsprung's disease or primary megacolon   *(1 mark)*
(ii) Absence of ganglion cells in nerve plexus of the large bowel wall, leading to spasm of the involved segment and dilatation of the normally innervated proximal loop   *(3 marks)*

(c) (i) Barium enema shows characteristic 'funnelling' at site of obstruction
Rectal biopsy for histological confirmation of absence of ganglion cells and/or cholinesterase staining for absence of acetylcholine   *(2 marks)*
(ii) Exclusion of the aganglionic segment by a 'pull-through' operation   *(2 marks)*

Comment

In Hirschsprung's disease there is a complete physiological obstruction in the distal colon at or above the peritoneal reflection. A barium enema is diagnostic and demonstrates the dilated normal proximal bowel leading to a coned transitional zone and the narrowed aganglionic zone. Those with a very short segment of aganglionic bowel may present later in childhood or, very occasionally, in adulthood.

Answer 8

(a) (i) Distended and tympanitic abdomen, minimally tender, with a possible palpable lesion
Increased bowel sounds
Empty rectum on rectal examination, with possible melaena on finger stall *(2 marks)*

(ii) Working diagnosis: subacute colonic obstruction caused by neoplasia or adhesions *(1 mark)*

(b) (i) Plain abdominal radiograph (supine and erect) *(1 mark)*

(ii) Features: dilated small and large bowel loops
Presence of air–fluid levels, faecal impaction and possibly the shadow of a colonic lesion
A barium enema should not be performed in large bowel obstruction *(2 marks)*

(c) Management:
FBC, U&Es, chest radiograph, ECG
Intravenous rehydration
Correct anaemia
Nil by mouth
Nasogastric aspiration if necessary
Catheterise to monitor urine output
Group and crossmatch
Intramuscular analgesia
Prepare for surgical relief of bowel obstruction
(4 marks)

Comment

In middle-aged and elderly people, a malignant colonic lesion must be suspected in the absence of a history of chronic constipation, inflammatory bowel disease and post-surgical adhesions. Obstructive symptoms are delayed in proximal colonic tumours, as a result of the liquid nature of their contents. These patients may, therefore, present late with anaemia and weight loss caused by tumour ulceration and invasion. Early diagnosis and appropriate surgical resection is curative in Duke's A and early B tumours. Some Duke's B and all C tumours require adjuvant chemotherapy. Preoperative radiotherapy may downstage the tumours in the treatment of rectal cancers.

Answer 9

(a) Idiopathic slow transit constipation
Laxative abuse
Irritable bowel syndrome
Obstructed defecation   *(2 marks)*

(b) Abdominal and digital rectal examination
Flexible sigmoidoscopy
Faecal occult bloods to screen for malignancy
Whole gut transit time using a capsule containing
radio-opaque markers
Defecating proctography – if main symptom is
difficulty in defecation   *(3 marks)*

(c) Wean patient off laxatives and counsel patient if there is
a pattern of laxative abuse
Prescribe bulk forming agents
Introduce bulk into diet
May require total colectomy if symptoms are
unremitting   *(5 marks)*

Comment

Chronic constipation is a common ailment of modern societies and tends to resolve with the introduction of high-fibre ingredients to the diet with bulk formers, such as Fybogel, Isogel, lactulose and normacol. Sedentary lifestyles predispose to this condition and physical activity should be encouraged. Idiopathic slow transit constipation may not respond to dietary or medical measures, and total colectomy and ileorectal anastomosis are curative in carefully selected patients. In those with difficulty in defecation with normal transit times, a feature is pelvic floor weakness which descends on straining. Other conditions are anterior rectocele and rectal intussusception; these patients may resort to digitally assisting defecation.

Answer 10

(a) Exacerbation of the diverticular disease
Acute diverticulitis *(2 marks)*

(b) Raised WBC
Raised CRP
If there is evidence of abscess formation, surgical drainage
Colonoscopy or barium enema following resolution to confirm diagnosis *(4 marks)*

(c) Bedrest
Intravenous fluids and nil by mouth
Intravenous Gram-negative anaerobe-sensitive antibiotics (metronidazole)
Colonoscopy/barium enema following resolution
Surgical resection of the involved segment if there is luminal narrowing as a result of scarring *(4 marks)*

Comment

Diverticulosis is the incidental finding of diverticula in the asymptomatic patient; diverticular disease is when patients have symptoms such as distension, flatulence and pelvic heaviness. Colonic segmentation in response to food may cause pain. Diverticulitis is inflammation of the diverticula, usually from inspissated faeces, and produces persistent lower abdominal pain and peritonism when there is serosal involvement. The sigmoid colon, which is most frequently involved, is palpable and tender. The aim of management is resolution of the infection and the exclusion of a concurrent colonic malignancy.

Answer 11

(a) (i) Digital rectal examination to palpate lesions in the rectum and pelvis
Rigid sigmoidoscopy to visualise the rectum and distal sigmoid colon
Protoscopy to visualise the anorectum   *(3 marks)*

   (ii) Carcinoma
Ulcerative colitis
Crohn's colitis
Polyps
Haemorrhoids   *(3 marks)*

(b) (i) Prolapsing haemorrhoids
(Other causes are anorectal polyps and mucosal prolapse)   *(1 mark)*

   (ii) Injection sclerotherapy
Rubber banding
Haemorrhoidectomy
Cryosurgery   *(3 marks)*

Comment

Rectal bleeding in any form should alert the clinician to the possibility of a large bowel tumour, especially in the older age group. The presence of piles (the most common cause of bleeding per rectum) should not preclude a sigmoidoscopic examination, because the piles may prove to be a red herring masking a more sinister proximal lesion. In the presence of a recent alteration in bowel habit with or without weight loss, imaging of the entire colon or colonoscopy may be required to exclude an occult neoplasm.

Answer 12

(a) Adenomatous
Inflammatory
Metaplastic
Harmatomatous   *(2 marks)*

(b) Endoscopic assessment of whether the lesion is benign
or malignant with multiple biopsies

Exclude the presence of polyps elsewhere in the colon

When the extent of the lesion makes it unsuitable for
endoscopic removal, surgical resection of the involved
segment of colon is advisable

Colonic surveillance follows treatment if indicated
(5 marks)

(c) This patient has, in all probability, adenomatous polyps
that may be familial or sporadic; familial polyposis
accounts for < 5% of the incidence; the remainder are
sporadic

Probable associated dietary factors are diets high in
animal fat and low in fibre   *(3 marks)*

Comment

Colonic polyps may be pedunculated or sessile; the risk of
malignant change increases with the increasing size of the polyp.
Polyps < 5 cm in size may be treated endoscopically by snaring or
diathermy obliteration. Large polyps, particularly when broad
based or sessile, may require surgical resection of the involved
segment of bowel. Polyps, with the exception of juvenile
metaplastic and inflammatory polyps, are prone to recur and these
patients must be kept under colonoscopic or imaging surveillance.

Answer 13

(a) (i) General appearance: size, shape, contact bleeding, punched out, shallow or irregular
Base: indurated or soft, fixed or mobile
Edges: everted, rolled up or sloping   *(3 marks)*

(ii) Multiple punch biopsies from the ulcer edge   *(2 marks)*

(b) (i) Liver   *(1 mark)*

(ii) Ultrasonography or CT scan of the liver   *(1 mark)*

(iii) Preoperative bowel preparation
An anterior resection of the rectum and distal sigmoid colon preserving the anal canal if the tumour is above the peritoneal reflection, or a synchronised combined abdominoperineal excision of the anorectum and distal sigmoid colon if the anal canal is involved   *(3 marks)*

Comment

It is necessary to counsel the patient about the planned operation and the need for either a temporary or permanent colostomy, its siting and management. Sphincter-preserving operations for rectal cancer aim at restoring bowel continuity, thereby avoiding a permanent stoma of an abdominoperineal excision. However, a 5cm distal clearance of the tumour must be attainable to avoid tumour recurrence at the anastomosis.

Answer 14

(a) (i) Ischiorectal abscess   *(1 mark)*

(ii) Anal mucosal crypt infection that persists to form a crypt abscess, which then enlarges and extends into perianal fat; expansion in the confined ischiorectal fossa leads to severe pain   *(3 marks)*

(b) (i) Fistula *in ano* *(1 mark)*

    (ii) Incision and drainage under a general anaesthetic with curettage of the abscess cavity with de-roofing
The cavity is packed with ribbon gauze soaked in antiseptic *(2 marks)*

    (iii) Low fistulous tracts are excised or laid open. In high fistulae, i.e. those that lie above the anal sphincters, a seton of nylon or braided wire is threaded in and tied gradually to obliterate the tract. Complicated or recurrent high fistulae may require excision, with preliminary faecal diversion *(3 marks)*

Comment

An ischiorectal abscess must be surgically drained on presentation. The presence of Gram-negative coliform organisms in the pus obtained suggests communication with the bowel and, rarely, biopsy of the abscess wall may reveal Crohn's disease. Medical treatment for Crohn's disease is then commenced and surgery limited to treating infective complications in the perineum. Persistent fistulae in the absence of inflammatory bowel disease are the result of recurrent perianal abscess formation and form tortuous tracts with multiple cutaneous openings. These may require staged surgical procedures for a cure, with a preliminary colostomy.

11 Urology

Answer 1

   (a) (i)   Hydronephrosis
            Cystic kidney
            Nephroblastoma (Wilms' tumour)
            Mesoblastic nephroma   *(2 marks)*
      (ii) Ultrasonography
            CT and/or MRI of the abdomen
            IVU
            Renal angiography   *(3 marks)*

   (b) (i)   Chest radiograph
            Liver scan
            Bone scan
            Bone marrow biopsy   *(2 marks)*
      (ii) Surgical: radical nephroureterectomy
            Radiotherapy: pre- and/or postoperative courses
            Chemotherapy: childhood tumours of the kidney
            or adjacent neuroectoderm are chemosensitive
            and respond well to a combination of two
            or more agents   *(3 marks)*

Comment

Nephroblastomas and neuroblastomas usually present as palpable
loin swellings with anaemia. Both lesions, as well as the rarer
mesoblastoma of the kidney, require radical excision.
Radiotherapy may be given before surgery to reduce the tumour
bulk, and a postoperative course is usual. Chemotherapy is usually
a combination of actinomycin D and vincristine or
cyclophosphamide and doxorubicin or cisplatin.

Answer 2

(a) Acute tubular necrosis
     Acute rejection
     Obstruction of the collecting system
     Infarction of transplant   *(2 marks)*

(b) Daily serum U&Es
     Isotope renography for state of perfusion
     Ultrasonography: reveals urinary tract obstruction,
     haematoma, urinoma and renal artery flow
     Percutaneous renal biopsy to diagnose acute tubular
     necrosis or acute rejection   *(3 marks)*

(c) (i)   Ciclosporin and/or azathioprine, anti-thymocyte
           globulin and prednisolone   *(2 marks)*
     (ii) Increased incidence of malignancies, i.e. with
           azathioprine immunosuppression, e.g. tumours of
           reticuloendothelial system, central nervous system
           and skin
           Increased incidence of upper GI bleeding
           with high doses of steroids   *(3 marks)*

Comment

Oliguria or anuria resulting from acute tubular necrosis occurs
immediately post-transplantation, with the extent of the tubular
damage dependent on the warm ischaemia time of the donor
kidney. Dialysis must be continued until the kidney recovers.
Rejection of the donor organ may be acute (within 3 months) or
chronic (thereafter), with progressive impairment of urine
production. The former responds favourably to anti-rejection
therapy.

Answer 3

(a) (i)   Pneumaturia   *(1 mark)*

     (ii)   Colovesical or colouteric fistula caused by invasion of either the urinary bladder or the ureter by either recurrent tumour or radiation damage   *(2 marks)*

(b) Intravenous urography
Cytoscopy
Cystourethrogram   *(3 marks)*

(c) Diverticular disease
Crohn's disease
Bladder cancer
Diabetes mellitus   *(4 marks)*

Comment

Fistulation into bladder or vaginal vault following adhesion to a diverticular inflammation of the colon, is excised with resection of the diseased bowel. Closure of the fistula is usually not feasible when it is caused by tumour infiltration or in the presence of post-irradiation fibrosis. Proximal defunctioning colostomy promotes healing following surgery and halts further contamination of the renal tract with bowel pathogens. It also facilitates further irradiation of the pelvis for tumour recurrence without the risk of radiation colitis.

Answer 4

(a) (i)   Pelviureteric colic caused by renal calculus disease   *(1 mark)*

     (ii)   Test urine for red blood cells   *(2 marks)*

(b) Adequate analgesia
Plain abdominal radiograph (KUB – kidneys, ureter and bladder) or a CT-KUB usually establishes the site of the calculus

Await spontaneous passage if calculus < 5 mm in size

An IVU and/or retrograde ureterogram followed by cystoscopic basket extraction if calculus > 5 mm in size

Cystoureterotomy if impacted in intravesical portion of distal ureter

Shock-wave lithotripsy or operative removal may be indicated for stones in the renal pelvis and proximal ureter   *(5 marks)*

(c) Hereditary and acquired defects in calcium and phosphate metabolism
Hyperparathyroidism
Hyperoxaluria
Cystinuria   *(2 marks)*

Comment

The need for open surgery for renal stones has been largely replaced by endoscopic or percutaneous extraction and extracorporeal shock-wave lithotripsy. Ureteric catheterisation and irrigation frequently dislodge impacted uteric calculi. Occasionally those impacted above the pelvic brim may be pushed up into the renal pelvis and fragmented or extracted percutaneously. N.B. Leaking abdominal aneurysms may mimic left-sided renal colic and are rapidly fatal unless promptly resuscitated and operated upon.

Answer 5

(a) Vesical calculus   *(2 marks)*

(b) Relieve retention by urethral catheter
Plain abdominal radiograph
Urethrocystoscopy or a cystogram and a
micturating urethrogram   *(4 marks)*

(c) Removal of the calculus by lithotripsy or
cystotomy   *(4 marks)*

Comment

Bladder stones are eight times more common in males than in females and are classified into primary and secondary stones. Chronic malnutrition in children is a predisposing factor for primary stones and chronic urinary infection for secondary stones. There may be a sense of incomplete emptying or interruption of the urinary stream with strangury. Urinary infection is a common presenting symptom.

Answer 6

    (a) Right reducible inguinal or femoral hernia
        Visible or tactile cough impulse above or below the
        inguinal ligament   *(3 marks)*

    (b) Prostatic enlargement or urethral stricture
        Palpable urinary bladder
        Enlarged prostate on per rectal examination or palpable
        stricture in penile urethra
        (3 marks)

    (c) Investigate urinary symptoms with flow studies
        Intravenous urography (IVU) and/or ultrasonography
        of urinary tract; urethrocystoscopy
        Treatment: prostatectomy or stricturoplasty and hernia
        repair   *(4 marks)*

Comment

Chronic increase in intra-abdominal pressure may precipitate an abdominal hernia. Chronic obstructive pulmonary disease, chronic constipation, ascites or an obstructive uropathy must be excluded in patients presenting with a groin hernia, and the precipitating cause(s) treated before the hernia is repaired.

Answer 7

(a) Haemorrhage from the prostatic bed with clot retention
Perforation of the urinary bladder   *(4 marks)*

(b) Myoadenomatous hyperplasia
Prostatic carcinoma   *(2 marks)*

(c) Bladder outflow obstruction leads to chronic retention
of urine, which produces hydronephrosis and atrophy
of the renal cortex, as a result of pressure effects and
infection
Prostatic cancer, when present (incidence 25% at
75 years of age), invades the capsule and may involve
the pelvis with bony metastases or the rectum
with fistula formation   *(4 marks)*

Comment

Haemorrhage after prostatic surgery is usually reactionary, leading to
clot retention, or secondary (usually a week after the operation) as a
result of infection or straining. Perforation of the bladder or
breaching the prostatic capsule may occur during transurethral
surgery and, if not immediately recognised, leads to severe
haemorrhage from the prostatic venous plexus in the latter. Bladder
perforation may be undetected postoperatively as a result of the
indwelling catheter preventing extravasation of urine. Both these
complications may require re-exploration under a general
anaesthetic.

Answer 8

(a) (i)   Testis, epididymis, cord structures
Tunica vaginalis, scrotal skin
Abdominal hernial contents   *(3 marks)*

(ii) Examination:
Get above it to exclude hernia
Palpate the testis and the epididymis on its upper
pole posteriorly; feel the cord structures and
examine for a hydrocele   *(2 marks)*

(b) (i) Teratoma, seminoma, yolk sac tumour *(3 marks)*
(ii) Orchidectomy
Radiotherapy to para-aortic nodes
Chemotherapy *(2 marks)*

Comment

Scrotal swellings include vaginal hydrocele (most common),
epididymal cyst, spermatocele, TB and tumour. Epididymo-
orchitis, caused by pyogenic organisms, generally has an acute
presentation. When a testicular tumour is suspected, percutaneous
biopsy is contraindicated because of seeding of tumour in the
needle track and spread to the groin nodes. An open biopsy with
frozen section histology should be performed, proceeding to
orchidectomy if malignancy is confirmed.

Answer 9

(a) (i) Torsion of the spermatic cord (testis) *(1 mark)*
(ii) Pyrexia; tender, swollen testis
Horizontal lie of testis ('dumb-bell sign')
Absent urethral discharge
Clear urine *(3 marks)*

(b) Surgical exploration with orchidopexy; if testis is
non-viable perform an orchidectomy
Fix the other testis to prevent it torting *(3 marks)*

(c) Exploration is no longer indicated due to testicular
non-viability
Antibiotics and analgesics
Observe in the ward until symptoms resolve
Testicular atrophy is the end result
The opposite testis must be fixed at an early date
(3 marks)

Comment

An attempt may be made to untwist a torted testis on presentation;
the immediate relief of pain indicates success. Surgical fixation
(orchidopexy) should then be performed without undue delay.

The opposite testis is also fixed, because the anatomical abnormality is likely to be bilateral.

Answer 10

  (a)   Diabetic neuropathy
         Psychosexual dysfunction
         Undescended testes
         Previous pelvic surgery or injury   *(3 marks)*

  (b)   Sperm count
         Sperm motility
         Percentage of normal to abnormal cells
         The pH and sugar content of seminal fluid   *(3 marks)*

  (c) (i)   Tuberculous epididymo-orchitis   *(1 mark)*
       (ii)   Urinalysis: microscopy and culture for
            tubercular bacilli
            Testicular biopsy for histological and
            microbiological evidence of TB   *(3 marks)*

Comment

An obvious cause of sterility is previous vasectomy and a request for surgical reversal is made on presentation. Surgical procedures for erectile dysfunction vary from penile revascularisation to the insertion of prosthetic implants.

Answer 11

  (a)   Urethral stricture
         Inflammatory: chronic urethritis (e.g. sexually
         transmitted infection)
         Traumatic: perineal injury producing partial rupture or
         ischaemic damage
         Iatrogenic: after urethral instrumentation or
         prostatic surgery in the older man   *(3 marks)*

  (b)   Urinary retention leads to bladder diverticula,
         hydroureter and hydronephrosis

Proximal urethral diverticulum leads to periurethral
abscess and urethral fistulae (watering can perineum)
Increased abdominal pressure of straining gives rise to
groin hernias, piles and rectal prolapse *(3 marks)*

(c) Intermittent urethral dilatation with gum-elastic
bougies, either separate or filiform, with screw-on
followers
Self-dilatation with soft Nelaton catheters
Urethrotomy under direct vision using an optical
urethrotome
Urethroplasty by excision of stricture and end-to-end
anastomosis or grafting after excision of more
extensive strictures *(4 marks)*

Comment

Gonococcal urethritis must be actively treated with antibiotics,
with the prevention of re-exposure. Ineffective treatment may lead
to spread of infection to produce posterior urethritis, prostatitis,
epididymo-orchitis or periurethral abscess. Dilatation of urethral
strictures may introduce infection, resulting in a bacteraemia
and/or septicaemia. Aseptic technique is, therefore, essential.
Contact tracing is an important public health measure.

Answer 12

(a) (i) Phimosis *(2 marks)*
    (ii) Inability to retract the foreskin, due to
         adhesions to the glans and scarring *(2 marks)*

(b) Balanitis
    Urethritis
    Cystitis *(3 marks)*

(c) Circumcision *(3 marks)*

Comment

True phimosis is scarring of the foreskin that does not retract without fissuring. A tight foreskin is what is usually encountered and is caused by physiological adhesions between the foreskin and glans. These may be gradually broken down by progressive freeing of the foreskin in the bath and retracting it over the glans. Failing this, dilatation of the foreskin under a short anaesthetic is effective. Circumcision is the preferred treatment for true phimosis and prevents balanitis, recurrent urinary infections and the slight long-term risk of penile cancer.

Answer 13

(a)	Ectopia vesicae	*(2 marks)*
(b)	Mucosa of the posterior bladder wall Trigone Ureteric orifices	*(3 marks)*
(c)	Absence of the umbilicus Groin hernias Separation and poor development of the pubic bones Epispadias in the male	*(2 marks)*
(d)	Treat urinary infection Assess and support renal function Surgical reconstruction of the bladder, abdominal wall and the pelvic ring (preliminary urinary diversion may be required)	*(3 marks)*

Comment

Ectopia vesicae results in the absence of the lower anterior abdominal wall, and the anterior bladder wall with the posterior bladder wall is fused to the margins of the abdominal wall defect. The quality of life is poor without treatment because of incontinence and recurrent urinary infections; there is also the long-term risk of bladder malignancy.

Answer 14

(a) Stress incontinence is caused by sphincter weakness and produces urinary leakage as a result of increased intra-abdominal pressure

Causes: weakness of distal sphincter mechanism combined with laxity of pelvic floor musculature as a result of complicated or neglected labour or multiple pregnancies

Neurogenic bladder dysfunction caused by demyelinating diseases (myelodysplasia, multiple sclerosis, syringomyelia) *(3 marks)*

(b) Exercise testing with 300 ml fluid in bladder and measure resulting fluid loss (of the order of 10–50 ml)

Urinary pressure–flow studies record bladder pressure and flow rate during micturition (distinguishes between genuine stress incontinence and detrusor instability) *(3 marks)*

(c) Minor degrees of stress incontinence can be controlled by improving the tone of the pelvic floor musculature with pelvic floor exercises

Surgical measures: colposuspension (suspending the vaginal fascia on either side of the bladder neck to the iliopubic ligaments)

Neurogenic bladder dysfunction may require implantation of a battery-operated urinary sphincter stimulator *(4 marks)*

Comment

It is important to distinguish stress incontinence from idiopathic detrusor muscle instability, because the outcome of surgery is significantly worse in the latter. The mainstay of treatment in the latter is the use of anticholinergic agents. Symptoms of stress incontinence as a result of neurogenic bladder dysfunction may progress to complete incontinence or retention as the disease progresses.

12

Vascular Surgery

Answer 1

(a) Diagnosis: acute limb ischaemia as a result of left common femoral arterial occlusion
Predisposing factors:
  Atrial fibrillation leading to embolism
  Thrombus on a previously diseased artery
  Aortic dissection *(3 marks)*

(b) Pallor and/or skin mottling
Cold, pulselessness and pain
Reduced skin sensation
Loss of function (toes cannot be moved)
Venous guttering *(3 marks)*

(c) Emergency surgical work-up:
  FBC, U&Es, chest radiograph, ECG, urethral catheterisation
  Group and crossmatch 4 units
Treat as acute or acute-on-chronic occlusion with systemic anticoagulation, arterial embolectomy or thrombectomy, with peroperative angiogram
In some instances thromboembolytic therapy may avoid surgery *(4 marks)*

Comment

Acute limb ischaemia is a surgical emergency. Systemic heparinisation (35 000–45 000 units/24 h) is commenced, and thromboembolectomy performed with a Fogarty balloon catheter. Occasionally, thrombolysis may be achieved with fibrinolytic agents, such as streptokinase or tissue plasminogen activator (tPA), which is infused intra-arterially. Long-term warfarin therapy must be started or the precipitating cause treated to prevent recurrence.

Answer 2

(a) (i) Peripheral vascular disease producing stenosis of the arteries of the right lower limb
Right common femoral artery or superficial and profunda femoral arteries   *(2 marks)*

(ii) Pathogenesis of atherosclerosis: adherent microthrombi and subintimal cholesterol deposits lead to atheromatous plaque formation and luminal narrowing; plaque haemorrhage leads to intimal ulceration; thrombi form on the ulcerated surface, giving rise to microemboli producing distal vessel occlusion   *(3 marks)*

(b) Smoking
Diabetes mellitus
Hypercholesterolaemia/high fat intake
Hypertension
Family history   *(2 marks)*

(c) Stop smoking
Close monitoring of diabetes/hypertension and response to treatment
Exercise to develop collateral circulation, weight reduction, low cholesterol diet
Foot care: podiatry/chiropody, protective footwear   *(3 marks)*

Comment

Claudication can usually be distinguished from musculoskeletal symptoms in the lower limb from the history of exercise-related pain. Peripheral vascular disease is generalised in nature, and the carotid arteries and aorta must be clinically assessed for occult lesions. The nutritional state of the affected foot, namely skin changes and ABPIs form part of the initial assessment.

Answer 3

(a) Pale, cold limb with loss of sensation, ischaemic skin changes
Reduced or absent femoral, popliteal, dorsalis pedis, posterior tibial
Reduced ABPIs
Neurological signs: reduced sensation, tone, power and reflexes with muscle wasting

(4 marks)

(b) (i) Retrograde transfemoral aortography   *(1 mark)*
(ii) Angioplasty of stenotic arterial lesions
Intra-arterial infusion of tPA at the site of stenosis through a radiologically positioned arterial catheter   *(2 marks)*

(c) Removal of arterial occlusive disease by endarterectomy
Bypass of occlusion using native vein or synthetic vascular grafts   *(3 marks)*

Comment

The presence of rest pain and ABPI > 0.5 suggest critical ischaemia. Pain usually involves the leg and foot, and there may be sensory or motor signs. Vascular reconstruction is usually required for limb salvage. However, in the presence of distal vessel disease, unresponsive to angioplasty or surgery, lumbar sympathectomy may improve skin perfusion.

Answer 4

(a)   Claudication or rest pain extending up to the buttock
Weak or absent distal pulses
Low resting and exercise ABPIs
Loss of muscle power   *(3 marks)*

(b)   (i)   Thrombosis, dislodgement of atheromatous plaque or intimal dissection during or after angioplasty producing arterial occlusion   *(2 marks)*

         (ii)   Analgesia; anticoagulation with intravenous heparin
Infusion of prostaglandin-derived thrombolytic agent (tPA)
Thromboembolectomy; repair or removal of intimal flap   *(3 marks)*

(c)   Smoking
Diabetes mellitus
Hyperlipidaemia/high fat intake
Hypertension
Family history   *(2 marks)*

Comment

Vascular imaging and interventional procedures are common in cardiology and vascular units. Complications arising therefrom, although uncommon, may require urgent surgical intervention. Patients who are admitted for these procedures must, therefore, be adequately assessed and prepared with informed consent for such eventualities.

Answer 5

(a) (i) False aneurysm of femoral artery   *(1 mark)*
    (ii) Duplex Doppler scan   *(1 mark)*
    (iii) By pressure occlusion with or without
          injection of a thrombotic agent into the
          sack; failing this, by surgical repair of
          arterial wall defect   *(2 marks)*

(b) (i) Thrombosis, embolus, intimal plaque
         formation, intimal dissection   *(2 marks)*
    (ii) Embolectomy/thrombectomy under
          imaging; intimal repair   *(4 marks)*

Comment

A false aneurysm is a pulsatile haematoma produced by bleeding
from the arterial puncture. Rarely, the adjacent femoral vein may
be injured, with the formation of a traumatic arteriovenous fistula.
This also presents as a pulsatile groin swelling. If detected early the
fistula may be closed off by pressure occlusion with a Doppler
probe. If allowed to mature it requires surgical repair. Fibrinolytic
therapy may lead to recanalisation after angiographic assessment
of the site of thrombotic arterial occlusion.

Answer 6

(a) (i) Abdominal aortic aneurysm   *(1 mark)*
    (ii) Atherosclerotic changes to vessel wall
          with intimal ulceration and destruction of
          elastic and muscle coats with intraluminal
          thrombus formation   *(2 marks)*

(b) Abdominal ultrasonography   *(1 mark)*
    Contrast-enhanced CT scan

(c) (i) Aneurysms < 6 cm in diameter and asymptomatic
– keep under surveillance
Aneurysms > 6 cm in diameter – inlay
of synthetic graft *(3 marks)*

(ii) Pre-operative work-up: chest radiograph, FBC
ECG
Renal function assessment
Hypertension control
Group and crossmatch 6–8 units blood *(3 marks)*

Comment

Abdominal aneurysms > 6 cm in diameter expand progressively over time, increasing the incidence of rupture or leakage. Elective surgery is aimed at obviating this risk, because survival after rupture is small. The chances of dying from rupture of aneurysms < 6 cm are the same as dying from elective aneurysectomy, so a conservative approach is followed, provided that the patient is kept under surveillance. Image-guided intraluminal grafting of aneurysms may obviate the need for open surgery.

Answer 7

(a) (i) Rupture of abdominal aortic aneurysm *(1 mark)*

(ii) Admit to HDU/ICU for preoperative optimisation
Maintain airway, administer O_2
Central and peripheral venous access
FBC and ABGs
Intravenous analgesia
Group and emergency crossmatch for 10–15 units blood
Monitor pulse, BP and respiration quarter-hourly
Volume replacement with crystalloids and plasma expanders, and with blood when available
Catheterise and monitor urine output
Inform the surgical and anaesthetic teams and operating theatre in preparation for emergency surgery

Chest and abdominal radiographs and ECG
Get consent from patient for emergency
abdominal surgery   (*3 marks*)

(b) Dacron graft replacement of ruptured
aortic aneurysm   (*1 mark*)

(c) (i)   Spontaneous retroperitoneal haemorrhage
as a result of over-anticoagulation   (*2 marks*)
(ii) Intravenous analgesia
Stop warfarin therapy
Resuscitation and replace blood volume
Administer coagulation factors in the form
of FFP and platelet concentrates   (*3 marks*)

Comment

It is vital to distinguish a ruptured or leaking aneurysm on
presentation, from left-sided pelviureteric colic or diverticulitis of
the left colon. Occasionally, retrosternal radiation of pain, coupled
with circulatory collapse, may simulate myocardial infarction. A
pulsatile and expansile abdominal mass and weak or absent
femoral pulses must be sought on examining the abdomen.
Surgical survival is determined largely by the duration of
hypotension (the interval between rupture and surgical control).
This determines the incidence of cardiorespiratory complications
and coagulation disorders in the postoperative period.

Answer 8

(a) (i) Stenosis of the right internal carotid
artery   *(1 mark)*

      (ii) Hypertension, diabetes mellitus, smoking,
hyperlipidaemia, family history   *(2 marks)*

(b) (i) Duplex scan of carotid vessels in the neck, or
bilateral carotid angiography   *(1 mark)*

      (ii) Site and extent of atheromatous carotid disease;
angiography provides additional information of
the intracranial arteries, and cross-perfusion
between the two hemispheres   *(2 marks)*

(c) Treat pre-existing cardiac disease and/or hypertension;
stop smoking
control diabetes mellitus
Treat hyperlipidaemia
Right carotid endarterectomy
Postoperatively systolic pressure to be kept
< 100 mmHg   *(4 marks)*

Comment

Atherosclerotic narrowing or ulceration is generally widespread
despite symptoms being confined to one anatomical region, supplied
by one or more diseased vessels. There is, therefore, the need to assess
the contralateral carotid supply, myocardial and renal function, and
the presence of other risk factors for stroke before planning surgery.

Answer 9

(a) Venous and vasculitic ulcers are caused by skin
breakdown, as a result of poor nutrition (trophic skin
changes)
Venous bleeding follows the erosion of the ulcer
into an adjacent or underlying varicosity   *(3 marks)*

(b) Tourniquets are to be avoided in first aid because they
cause venous congestion and increased blood loss; they
cause arterial damage if applied too tightly

CHAPTER 12 – ANSWERS

Venous haemorrhage is readily controlled by
elevation of the affected limb and a local pressure
dressing   *(3 marks)*

(c)   Control local oedema by graduated support stockings
or limb elevation
Topical ulcer treatment with 4-layer bandaging until
healing is complete
Surgical removal of the underlying varices   *(4 marks)*

Comment

It is important to ensure venous ulcer healing before proceeding to
varicose vein surgery. Tourniquets can cause exsanguination by
preventing venous outflow but not arterial inflow. Tourniquets
tight enough to occlude the latter may cause vascular damage and
thrombosis. Nerve conduction injury may also occur and, if
applied for a number of hours, may produce muscle necrosis and
precipitate renal failure. Arterial tourniquet is used for some
surgical procedures, but should not be left in place for more than
an hour.

Answer 10

(a)   (i)   Venous or stasis ulcer caused by trophic skin
changes and underlying venous stasis   *(1 mark)*
(ii) Indolent, shallow and moist granulating floor
with associated varicosities and surrounding
pigmentation
Induration and pitting oedema results in
poor skin nutrition   *(2 marks)*

(b)   (i)   Limb elevation; wound toilet and non-stick
dressing and 4-layer bandaging
Split-skin grafting if required   *(2 marks)*
(ii) Treat the associated varicose veins surgically
after healing of ulcer   *(1 mark)*

(c)   Ischaemic ulcers: caused by poor tissue perfusion as a result of pressure (decubitus ulcers), atherosclerotic or diabetic vascular occlusive disease

Neuropathic ulcers are anaesthetic and caused by peripheral nerve degeneration, as in leprosy and diabetic neuritis

Tropical ulcers are the result of chronic skin infections caused by bacteria (*Mycobacterium ulcerans* in Buruli ulcer) or fungi (actinomycosis, mycetoma)

(4 marks)

Comment

Ulcers caused by vascular diseases are painful, the exceptions being pressure ulcers and diabetic ulcers where nerve damage occurs alongside the ischaemic changes.

Venous ulcers in the leg may extend and become circumferential, thereby endangering the viability of the limb. Chronicity may give rise to squamous cell carcinoma (Marjolin's ulcer); a biopsy should be undertaken when in doubt.

Answer 11

(a)   Increase in body temperature and pulse
Increase in limb diameter and warmth
Tenderness on palpation, with or without induration
Positive Homans' sign   *(3 marks)*

(b)   (i)   Deep vein thrombosis (DVT) of calf and/or thigh   *(1 mark)*
      (ii)   Venous stasis leads to the following sequence: DVT, pulmonary embolus, fall in pulmonary arterial pressure, with consequent fall in gaseous exchange, fall in cardiac output and cardiac arrest   *(3 marks)*

    (c)   Management of DVT:
Colour flow duplex imaging confirms DVT and its
proximal extent (venogram gives further information
on the iliac veins)
Intravenous heparin infusion of 30 000–40 000 IU/24 h
Commence long-term warfarin therapy before
discharge; monitor anticoagulation profile
periodically   *(3 marks)*

Comment

In young patients, in addition to known risk factors, such as oral
contraception and smoking, spontaneous venous thrombosis may
be associated with deficiencies in the coagulation profile, i.e.
protein C, protein S and anti-thrombin III. Prolonged immobility
in healthy adults or during long-haul flights, may predispose to
DVT. Thrombosis of the common femoral vein with an associated
lymphangitis produces a very swollen 'white leg' (phlegmasia alba
dolens); extensive thrombosis of the iliac and pelvic veins
produces venous obstruction and a 'blue leg' (phlegmasia caerulea
dolens). In the latter, venous gangrene may threaten limb viability.

Answer 12

    (a)   (i)   Pulmonary embolus   *(1 mark)*
          (ii)   ECG
                Ventilation–perfusion scan
                ABGs   *(2 marks)*

    (b)   Resuscitation
Analgesia
Systemic anticoagulation
Swan–Ganz catheterisation to measure pulmonary
artery wedge pressure and for selective thrombolysis
Surgical embolectomy if cardiorespiratory function
deteriorates   *(5 marks)*

(c) Stop smoking; avoid oral contraception
Compression stockings
Early mobilisation
Heparin prophylaxis   *(2 marks)*

Comment

Pulmonary emboli originate from thrombus in the veins of the pelvis or lower limbs. The latter may give rise to local symptoms and/or signs and signal an impending catastrophe. Deep venous thrombosis must, therefore, be actively treated with immediate systemic anticoagulation. Thrombosis in pelvic veins extending to the inferior vena cava may require angiographic placement of a filter above it to prevent embolisation.

13

ICU & Anaesthesia

Answer 1

(a) i. Cerebral hypoxia/hypotension
ii. Hypoglycaemia
iii. Sepsis or toxins
iv. Anaesthetic and other drugs
v. Head injury   *(4 marks)*

(b) Evaluation of a confused patient is performed as follows:
- Assessment of neurological state by verbal stimulae – awake, coherent patients are asked what is troubling them
- Nursing notes and team discussion may identify dysfunctional sleep patterns or inadequate analgesia
- Exclude withdrawal syndrome, pre-eclampsia
- Determine O_2 saturation, if < 90% suggests a hypoxic aetiology
- Low BP and urine output suggest CNS hypoperfusion
- Fever and tachycardia suggest sepsis or delirium tremens
- Neck stiffness and up going plantar reflexes suggest meningitis, although the latter may be difficult to demonstrate in an agitated patient
- Focal findings on neurologic examination suggest stroke, haemorrhage, or increased intracranial pressure (ICP).   *(3 marks)*

   (c)   Treatment of a confused and agitated patient may involve one or all of the following steps:

- Underlying causes (eg, hypoxia, shock, drugs) should be addressed
- The environment should be optimized (eg, darkness, quiet, and minimal sleep interruption at night) as much as is compatible with medical care
- Family presence, soothing auditory stimulae (music) and consistent nursing personnel may be calming
- Pharmacologic treatment is dictated by the prime symptoms. Pain is treated with analgesics; anxiety and insomnia, with sedatives; and psychosis and delirium, with small doses of an antipsychotic drug
- Intubation and ventilation may be needed to alleviate increased respiratory effort or when sedative and analgesic requirements jeopardise the airway or respiratory drive   *(3 marks)*

Comment

ICU patients may be agitated, confused, and in discomfort and occasionally become frankly psychotic (ICU psychosis). These symptoms may interfere with patient care and safety and may become life threatening (eg, the patient dislodges his endotracheal tube or IV lines).

The ICU environment may exacerbate the problem; constant monitoring and noise levels and bright lights, result in sleep deprivation. The elderly are particularly vulnerable and patients with relatively normal mentation commonly experience fear and uncertainty of outcome.

Answer 2

(a) Stress ulceration   *(1 mark)*

(b) Stress ulceration in critically ill patients is caused by ischaemic injury to the gastric mucosa, loss of cytoprotectants and the disruption of the gastric mucosal barrier to acid injury   *(2 marks)*

(c) The major risk factors are respiratory failure, coagulopathy, sepsis, hypotension and hepatic and renal failure   *(3 marks)*

(d) The prevention of stress ulceration has focused on reducing the quantity of luminal acid, using H2 receptor antagonists or proton pump inhibitors. The overall objective of such therapy is to increase the pH of the stomach above 3.5 with cimetidine, ranitidine, omeprazole, cesomeprazole or lansoprazole   *(2 marks)*

(e) Nosocomial pneumonia is common in critically ill patients, and remains the leading cause of death. It has been established that the use of anti-acid therapy promotes gastric colonization with pathogenic bacteria, and that aspiration of these bacteria may cause nosocomial pneumonia. The use of ranitidine or omeprazole is associated with a higher incidence of nosocomial pneumonia compared to sucralfate   *(2 marks)*

Comment

Patients with major gastroduodenal bleeds have a high mortality, and, consequently, prophylaxis against this complication has become a central issue in ICU care.

Stress ulceration is a gastrointestinal mucosal injury related to critical illness. The ulceration may vary from errosive gastritis to deep haemorrhaging ulcerations. There is a relationship between severity of illness and incidence of ulceration. The development of stress ulceration may not be related to a history of peptic ulcer disease or Helicobacter infection. The cause is multifactorial, and related to hypoperfusion and loss of host defenses. The development of clinically significant bleeding compounds the management of the critically ill patient, due to loss of physiological reserve and acute hypovolaemia and end organ injury. The mortality rate is high varying between 48.5% and 87.5%.

Answer 3

(a) Internal jugular vein, external jugular vein, subclavian vein, femoral vein, and venous cutdown on the basilic vein. The choice of site depends on whether a peripheral or central vein cannulation is required, depending on the nutrients and the duration of infusion   *(3 marks)*

(b) The patient's coagulation status and platelet count should be normalised before CVC insertion. The area must be sterile and the line inserted using full aseptic technique   *(2 marks)*

(c) The following precautions are essential in the management of CVCs:
- After a subclavian or internal jugular catheter is inserted, a chest radiograph is taken to locate the catheter tip and to exclude a pneumothorax
- To prevent cardiac arrhythmias, catheters in the right atrium or ventricle should be withdrawn until the tip is within the superior vena cava
- The catheter may be tunnelled through the subcutaneous tissue before venous entry to reduce catheter associated infection
- The skin entry site must be cleansed and inspected daily for local infection; the catheter must be replaced if local or systemic infection occurs
- Tunnelled catheters may be left for long periods and should incorporate a 'heplock', a heparin solution in the lumen to prevent catheter blockage   *(2 marks)*

(d)   Pneumothorax, accidental arterial cannulation, sepsis

(3 marks)

Comment

Patients needing secure or long-term vascular access (eg, for administration of antibiotics, chemotherapy, or TPN) are best treated with a tunnelled central venous catheter (CVC). CVCs allow infusion of solutions that are too concentrated or irritating for peripheral veins and also allow monitoring of central venous pressure. CVCs are inserted using sterile technique and local anesthesia. CVC may be inserted peripherally 'PIC' line if the infused solutions are non-irritant.

Percutaneous femoral lines must be inserted below the inguinal ligament. Otherwise, laceration of the external iliac vein or artery above the inguinal ligament may result in retroperitoneal hemorrhage; external compression of these vessels is nearly impossible. The subclavian vein also is not compressible with external pressure, and thus hemorrhage can be serious. A cutdown decreases the risk of bleeding-associated complications, particularly if coagulopathy is present.

Pneumothorax occurs in 1% of patients after CVC insertion. Atrial or ventricular arrhythmias frequently occur during catheter insertion but are generally self-limited and subside when the guide wire or catheter is withdrawn from within the heart. The incidence of catheter bacterial colonization without systemic infection may be as high as 35%, whereas that of true sepsis is 2 to 8%. Accidental arterial catheterisation may rarely require surgical repair of the artery. Hydrothorax and hydromediastinum may occur when catheters are positioned extravascularly. Catheter damage to the tricuspid valve, bacterial endocarditis, and air and catheter embolism occur rarely.

Answer 4

(a) Swan-Ganz catheter, also called pulmonary artery catheter (PAC), is a balloon-tipped, flow-directed catheter that is inserted via central veins through the right side of the heart into the pulmonary artery. The catheter typically contains several ports that can monitor pressure or inject fluids   *(2 marks)*

(b) The PAC is inserted through the subclavian or internal jugular vein with the balloon deflated. Once the catheter tip reaches the superior vena cava, partial inflation of the balloon permits blood flow to guide the catheter. The position of the catheter tip is usually determined by pressure monitoring or occasionally by fluoroscopy. Entry into the right ventricle is indicated by a sudden increase in systolic pressure to about 30 mm Hg; diastolic pressure remains unchanged from right atrial or vena caval pressure. When the catheter enters the pulmonary artery, the systolic pressure does not change, but diastolic pressure rises above right ventricular end-diastolic pressure or central venous pressure (CVP), ie, the pulse pressure narrows. Further movement of the catheter wedges the balloon in a distal pulmonary artery. A chest radiograph confirms appropriate placement   *(3 marks)*

(c) Data from PACs are used mainly to determine cardiac output and pulmonary artery occlusion pressure (equivalent to preload also termed pulmonary capillary wedge pressure). Other variables can be calculated from the cardiac output. These include systemic and pulmonary vascular resistance and right and left ventricular stroke work. Some PACs also include a sensor to measure central (mixed) venous O_2 saturation   *(3 marks)*

(d) Pulmonary artery perforation, cardiac arrhythmias   *(2 marks)*

Comment

A pulmonary artery catheter is rarely used – except perhaps in cardiac surgery. Most physicians believe PACs aid in the management of certain critically ill patients when combined with other objective and clinical data. PACs have not been shown to reduce morbidity and mortality. Indeed, PAC use has been associated with increased mortality. This finding may be explained by complications of PAC use and misinterpretation of the data obtained.

PACs may be difficult to insert. Cardiac arrhythmias are the most common complication. Pulmonary infarction secondary to overinflated or permanently wedged balloons, pulmonary artery perforation, intracardiac perforation, valvular injury, and endocarditis may occur. Rarely, the catheter may curl into a knot within the right ventricle (especially in patients with heart failure, cardiomyopathy, or increased pulmonary pressure).

Pulmonary artery rupture occurs in < 0.1% of PAC insertions. This catastrophic complication is often fatal and occurs immediately upon wedging the catheter–either initially or on subsequent occlusion pressure check. Because of this, many physicians prefer to monitor pulmonary artery diastolic pressures rather than occlusion pressures.

Answer 5

(a) Sepsis is systemic infection accompanied by the systemic inflammatory response syndrome (SIRS)

(1 mark)

(b) Systemic inflammatory response syndrome (SIRS) represents an acute inflammatory reaction with systemic manifestations caused by release into the bloodstream of numerous endogenous mediators of inflammation   *(2 marks)*

(c) Acute pancreatitis, major trauma, burns   *(3 marks)*

(d)   Severe sepsis is accompanied by signs of failure of at least one organ. Cardiovascular failure is typically manifested by hypotension, respiratory failure by hypoxemia, renal failure by oliguria, and haematologic failure by coagulopathy   *(1 mark)*

(e)   An inflammatory stimulus (eg, a bacterial toxin) triggers production of proinflammatory mediators, including tumour necrosis factor and interleukin-1 (IL-1). These cytokines cause neutrophil-endothelial cell adhesion, activate the clotting mechanism, and generate microthrombi. They also release numerous other mediators, including leukotrienes, lipoxygenase, histamine, bradykinin, serotonin, and IL-2.   These are opposed by anti-inflammatory mediators, such as IL-4 and IL-10, resulting in a negative feedback mechanism.

Initially, arteries and arterioles dilate, decreasing peripheral arterial resistance. Cardiac output typically increases during this stage referred to as "warm shock." Later, cardiac output may decrease, blood pressure falls (with or without an increase in peripheral resistance), and typical features of shock appear. Decreased perfusion causes dysfunction and sometimes failure of one or more organs – kidneys, lungs, liver, brain and heart. Coagulopathy may develop because of intravascular coagulation with consumption of major clotting factors   *(3 marks)*

Comment

Severe sepsis, and septic shock are inflammatory states resulting from systemic bacterial infection. They are accompanied by SIRS. SIRS has previously been defined by 2 or more of the following:

- Temperature $> 38°$ C or $< 36°$ C
- Heart rate > 90 beats/min
- Respiratory rate > 20 breaths/min or $Paco_2 < 32$ mm Hg
- WBC count $> 12,000$ cells/μL or < 4000 cells/μL, or $> 10\%$ immature forms

However, these criteria are now viewed as suggestive but not sufficiently precise to be diagnostic.

In severe sepsis and septic shock, there is critical reduction in tissue perfusion. Common causes include gram-negative organisms, staphylococci and meningococci. Symptoms often begin with shaking chills and include fever, hypotension, oliguria, and confusion. Acute failure of multiple organs can occur, including the lungs, kidneys and liver. Treatment is aggressive fluid resuscitation, antibiotics, supportive care and sometimes intensive control of blood glucose, and administration of corticosteroids and activated protein C.

Answer 6

(a) Malignant hyperthermia *(1 mark)*

(b) Halothane, a once popular but now rarely used volatile anaesthetic, has been linked to a large proportion of cases, however, all halogenated volatile anaesthetics are potential triggers of malignant hyperthermia. Succinylcholine, a neuromuscular blocking agent, is also a trigger for malignant hyperthermia *(2 marks)*

(c) Malignant hyperthermia is caused in a large proportion (50–70%) of cases by a mutation of the ryanodine receptor type 1 (RYR1), located on the sarcoplasmic reticulum, the organelle within the skeletal muscle cells that stores calcium. RYR1 opens in response to increases in intracellular Ca^{2+} level mediated by L-type calcium channels, thereby resulting in a drastic increase in intracellular calcium levels and muscle contraction. RYR1 has two sites believed to be important for reacting to changing Ca^{2+} concentrations: the A-site and the I-site. The A-site is a high affinity Ca^{2+} binding site that mediates RYR1 opening. The I-site is a lower affinity site that mediates the protein's closing. Caffeine, halothane, and other triggering agents act by drastically increasing the affinity of the A-site for Ca^{2+} and concomitantly decreasing the affinity of the I-site in mutant proteins. Mg^{2+} also affect RYR1 activity, causing the protein to close by acting at either the A- or I-sites. In malignant hyperthermia mutant proteins, the affinity for Mg^{2+} at either or these sites is greatly reduced. The end result of these alterations is greatly increased Ca^{2+} release due to a lowered activation and heightened deactivation threshold. The process of reabsorbing this excess Ca^{2+} consumes large amounts of adenosine triphosphate(ATP), the main cellular energy carrier, and generates the excessive heat (hyperthermia) that is the hallmark of the disease. The muscle cell is damaged by the depletion of ATP and possibly the high temperatures, and cellular constituents leak into the circulation, including potassium, myoglobin, creatine and creatine kinase   (3 marks)

(d) The current treatment of choice is the intravenous administration of dantrolene, discontinuation of triggering agents, and supportive therapy directed at correcting hyperthermia, acidosis, and organ dysfunction. Treatment must be instituted rapidly on clinical suspicion of the onset of malignant hyperthermia. Dantrolene is a muscle relaxant that works directly on the ryanodine receptor to prevent the release of calcium   (4 marks)

Comment

Malignant hyperthermia is typically a fulminant life-threatening disease, also referred to as a syndrome, which occurs when a person with malignant hyperthermia susceptibility trait is exposed to triggering factors, which include most inhalational anaesthetics, succinylcholine and, rarely, stress.

Classic malignant hyperthermia is characterised by hypermetabolism, muscle rigidity, muscle injury and increased sympathetic nervous system activity. Hypermetabolism, reflected by elevated carbon dioxide production, precedes the increase in body temperature.

The incidence has been reported to be between 1:4,500 to 1:60,000 procedures involving general anaesthesia. This disorder occurs

CHAPTER 13 – ANSWERS

worldwide and affects all racial groups. Most cases however occur in children and young adults.

Malignant hyperthermia is often inherited as an autosomal dominanat disorder, for which there are at least 6 loci of interest. Malignant hyperthermia is phenotypically and genetically related to central core disease, an autosomal dominant disorder characterised both by malignant hyperthermia symptoms and myopathy.

Answer 7

(a) The indications for endotracheal intubation include:
- Failure to protect the airway
- Failure to maintain the airway
- Failure of ventilation
- Failure of oxygenation
- Anticipated clinical deterioration (eg, expanding neck haematoma) and/or impending need for surgical intervention *(3 marks)*

(b) The contraindications for endotracheal intubation include:
- Absolute
  Upper airway obstruction
  Loss of facial landmarks
- Relative
  Anticipated difficult airway
  Failed intubation *(2 marks)*

(c) The complications of endotracheal intubation include:
- Right mainstem intubation
- Oesophageal intubation
- Dental trauma
- Pneumothorax
- Post-intubation pneumonia
- Vocal cord avulsion
- Failure to intubate
- Hypotension *(3 marks)*

(d)   RSI is an organised approach to endotracheal
        intubation comprising specific steps and actions
        leading to rapid sedation and paralysis with (ideally) no
        positive pressure ventilation. The purpose is to achieve
        optimal and rapid tracheal intubation in patients who
        are at risk for aspiration, that is, any patient who
        presents to the Emergency department   *(2 marks)*

Comment

Endotracheal intubation may be performed in any clinical setting
in which the appropriate equipment, including a ventilator,
medications, and trained personnel are available. The procedure
may be indicated in cardiac arrest, sepsis, airway obstruction,
multiple trauma, closed head injury when the patient is having
difficulty maintaining a patent airway, problems with ventilation
or oxygenation, or an anticipated deterioration of the patient's
condition. Except for defibrillation in witnessed pulseless loss of
consciousness, tracheal intubation is the first procedure
performed on a critically ill patient with respiratory insufficiency
or respiratory failure.

In the Emergency Department setting, patients are typically
endotracheally intubated using a specific protocol known as rapid
sequence intubation (RSI). Unlike in the preoperative setting, in
which the patient has fasted for a minimum of 6–8 hours before
the procedure, patients who need emergent intubation are
assumed to have a full stomach. The key point in RSI is to *not* assist
ventilation (eg, bag-valve-mask ventilation) of the patient for
continued oxygenation after the administration of paralytic
medications to avoid insufflation of the stomach, leading to
regurgitation of stomach contents and possible aspiration.

With adequate preoxygenation preceding paralysis, desaturation is
avoided during RSI despite a period of apnoea. In healthy adult
volunteers who have been preoxygenated for 3–5 minutes, the
average time to desaturation (defined as an oxygen saturation
<90%) is approximately 8 minutes. A patient in critical condition
with respiratory compromise may have significantly less reserve.

CHAPTER 13 – ANSWERS

Answer 8

(a) Physiological changes during inflation include:
  - Increased systemic blood pressure, central venous pressure and heart rate
  - Increased blood volume (up to 15%)
  - Reduction in the capacitance of the vascular bed
  - Temperature reduction in the non-perfused limb
  - Production of anaerobic metabolites *(3 marks)*

(b) Physiological changes during deflation include:
  - Reperfusion of limb with reduction in blood volume and systemic vascular resistance leading to decreased blood pressure, central venous pressure and heart rate
  - Reduction in core temperature
  - Mixed acidosis with decreased pO_2 and pH, while increased pCO_2, K^+ and free radicals
  - Rebound hyper-reperfusion *(3 marks)*

(c) Applying a pressurised pneumatic cuff (tourniquet) to a limb can be used to prevent the central spread of local anaesthetic during intravenous regional anaesthesia. It may also be used to reduce bleeding and improve the surgical field when operating on an exsanguinated limb *(2 marks)*

(d) The incidence of complications is related to the inflation pressure and the duration of inflation. Important complications include:
  - Limb ischaemia
  - Local anaesthetic toxicity
  - Pressure-related nerve damage
  - Damage to underlying vessels, increasing the incidence of microemboli formation in the exsanguinated limb
  - Tourniquet pain
  - Hypertension *(2 marks)*

Comment

Surgical tourniquets prevent blood flow to a limb and enable surgeons to work in a bloodless operative field. This allows surgical procedures to be performed with improved precision, safety and speed. Tourniquets are widely used in orthopaedics and plastic surgery, as well as in intravenous regional anesthesia (Bier block anaesthesia) where they serve the additional function of preventing local anesthetic in the limb from entering general circulation.

Despite many advances in tourniquet technology, tourniquet related injuries continue to be of concern. High pressures under a tourniquet cuff can cause nerve, muscle and skin injury. Minimising tourniquet pressure, reducing inflation time and using a microprocessor-controlled pneumatic tourniquet, and allows pressure to be accurately monitored and controlled, reduces the risk of tourniquet related injury.

Answer 9

(a) Epidurals may be used:
- For analgesia alone, where surgery is not contemplated. An epidural for pain relief (eg, in childbirth) is unlikely to cause loss of muscle power, but is not usually sufficient for surgery
- As an adjunct to general anaesthesia. The anaesthetist may use epidural analgesia in addition to general anaesthesia. This may reduce the patient's requirement for opioid analgesics
- As a sole technique for surgical anaesthesia, usually with sedation. Some operations, most frequently Caesarian section, may be performed using an epidural anaesthetic as the sole technique. Typically the patient would remain awake during the operation. The dose required for anaesthesia is much higher than that required for analgesia

- For post-operative analgesia, in the above situations. Analgesics are given into the epidural space for a few days after surgery, provided a catheter has been inserted
- For the treatment of back pain. Injection of analgesics and steroids into the epidural space may improve some forms of back pain

(4 marks)

(b) Contraindications for epidural technique include:
- Patient refusal
- Bleeding disorder (coagulopathy) or anticoagulant medication (eg, warfarin)
- Infection near the point of insertion
- Septicaemia or bacteraemia
- Hypovolaemia   *(3 marks)*

(c) Three complications of epidural technique include:
- Hypotension
- Block failure
- Accidental dural puncture   *(3 marks)*

Comment

Epidural anaesthesia is a form of regional anaesthesia involving injection of drugs through a catheter placed into the epidural space. The injection can cause both a loss of sensation and a loss of pain (analgesia), by blocking the transmission of pain signals through nerves in or near the spinal cord. Hypotension is the most common complication of epidural technique. A systolic blood pressure of less than 100 mmHg, or a fall of greater than 30% should be considered significant. Hypotension usually results from the physiologic effects of sympathetic blockade on the cardiovascular system. The incidence of hypotension can be markedly reduced by the employment of preventive measures such as intravenous pre-loading and vasopressor therapy.

Answer 10

(a)   Opioid analgesics, gastroparesis   *(2 marks)*

(b)   Wound disruption, aspiration of gastric contents
                                                        (2 marks)

(c)   The final common pathway for efferent responses that
      produce emesis (vomiting) is the vomiting centre,
      which controls the act of vomiting. Numerous
      neuronal pathways converge on the vomiting centre in
      the medulla where the vomiting reflex is initiated. The
      vomiting centre is not a discrete anatomical site, but
      represents inter-related neuronal networks. Inputs to
      the vomiting centre include vagal sensory pathways
      from the gastro-intestinal tract and neuronal pathways
      from the labyrinths, higher centres of the cortex,
      intracranial pressure receptors and the chemoreceptor
      trigger zone (CTZ). The CTZ in the area prostrema of
      the 4th ventricle of the brain acts as the entry point for
      emetic stimuli and humoral substances. The CTZ is
      outside the blood-brain barrier and therefore responds
      to stimuli from either the cerebrospinal fluid or the
      blood. When activated the vomiting centre induces
      vomiting via stimulation of the salivary and respiratory
      centres and the pharyngeal, gastrointestinal and
      abdominal muscles. A wide variety of
      neurotransmitters including histamine, acetylcholine,
      dopamine, noradrenaline, adrenaline,
      5–Hydroxytryptamine (5HT) and Substance P have a
      role in the genesis of vomiting. In support of their role
      in vomiting, it has been shown that antagonists of
      receptors for each of these transmitters have
      anti-emetic effects   *(3 marks)*

(d) The management of patients with postoperative nausea and vomiting is aimed at:
- Identification and elimination of the underlying cause where possible
- Control of the symptoms if it is not possible to eliminate the underlying cause
- Correction of electrolyte, fluid or nutritional deficiencies
- A wide range of drugs has been shown to have effects on nausea and vomiting. These include antihistamines, anticholinergics, dopamine receptor antagonists, 5–HT$_3$ receptor antagonists, cannabinoids, benzodiazepines, corticosteroids and gastroprokinetic agents. Each of the drugs affects different receptors, and some act at a number of different sites. Mutli-drug approach is more effective than single drug therapy

It is important to care for the wellbeing and comfort of the patient, since poor management of this can lead to delayed recovery, poor clinical outcome and aversion to future treatment. *(3 marks)*

Comment

Post-operative nausea and vomiting (PONV) is one of the most common side effects associated with surgical procedures. It can be very distressing for patients, can lead to medical complications which include possible wound disruption, oesophageal tears, gastric herniation, muscular fatigue, dehydration and electrolyte imbalance. There is also an increased risk of pulmonary aspiration of vomitus. Apart from the medical complications, PONV can have psychological effects that may result in patients experiencing anxiety about undergoing further surgery. The cost implications of PONV are due to delayed recovery and discharge, increased medical care and occasionally reoperation.

In the UK, it has been estimated that PONV affects between one and two million patients every year. Risk factors for PONV can be divided into patient risk factors, procedural risk factors, anaesthetic risk factors and postoperative risk factors.

Patient risk factors

Certain patient groups are at a higher risk of PONV than others. The following are some of the particular risk factors.

- **Gender**. The prevalence of PONV is three times higher in women than in men. This gender difference is not evident in pre-pubertal children or in the elderly, which indicates that there may be hormonal involvement
- **Age**. Children are twice as likely to develop PONV than adults. PONV is low in very young children, increases up to the age of 5 and is highest in children between the ages of 6 and 16 years
- **Obesity**. Fat-soluble anaesthetics may accumulate in adipose tissue and continue to be released for an extended period resulting in prolonged side effects, including PONV
- **Migraine**. Patients with a history of migraine are more likely to experience PONV
- **Pre-operative eating patterns**. Adequate preoperative fasting reduces the risk of PONV, whereas excessive starvation appears to increase the risk. In emergency surgery, where there has not been an adequate fast, the risk is increased
- **History of PONV or motion sickness**. Such patients may have a lower threshold to nausea and vomiting than the rest of the population. Anxiety, due to a previous experience of PONV, may add to the risk
- **Gastroparesis**. Patients with delayed gastric emptying secondary to an underlying disease may be at increased risk of PONV

Procedural risk factors

The type and duration of surgery is a major factor in PONV. Extended surgical procedures are more likely to lead to PONV than shorter operations, and the following surgical procedures predispose to a higher incidence of PONV.

- **Gynaecological**
- **Abdominal, especially gastrointestinal**
- **Laparoscopic**
- **Ear, Nose and Throat**
- **Ophthalmic**

Anaesthetic risk factors

Certain anaesthetic agents have been associated with a higher incidence of PONV these include:

- Choice of premedication
- Use of opioid analgesics
- Use of nitrous oxide
- Use of some inhalation agents
- Longer procedures and greater depth of anaesthesia

Post-operative risk factors

A number of post-operative factors can influence the risk of PONV.

- **Pain** – relief of pain is often associated with the relief of nausea, though the use of opioid analgesics may exacerbate the risk because of their known emetic potential. However some patients may be willing to tolerate a degree of pain provided they are free of nausea and vomiting
- **Dizziness** – PONV is increased in patients who experience dizziness.
- **Early ambulation** - Early or sudden movement can increase the risk of PONV, especially if the patients have received opioids
- **Use of opioids** – the use of opioids may exacerbate the risk of PONV because of their known emetic potential
- **Hypotension** – postoperative hypotension is common and can trigger PONV
- **Premature oral intake** – It is generally considered wise to restrict oral intake, and then to recommend small sips of water to minimise the risk of PONV

No single drug or class of drug is fully effective in controlling PONV, presumably because none block all pathways to the vomiting centre. However, because of the multi-receptor origin of PONV, combination therapy is being more widely employed. The table below summarises commonly used antiemetics.

Class	Drug
Anti-cholinergic	scopolamine (L-hyoscine)
Anti-histamine	cinnarizine cyclizine promethazine
Dopamine antagonists	metoclopramide domperidone droperidol (withdrawn 2001) haloperidol
Cannabinoid	nabilone
Corticosteroid	dexamethasone
Histamine analogue	betahistine
$5HT_3$-receptor antagonist	granisetron ondansetron tropisetron

PART THREE

Essay Writing

14

Structured Outlines

Question 1

Write an essay on the diagnosis and treatment of primary skin cancers.

Plan

Types of skin cancer:
  Basel cell cancer
  Melanoma
  Squamous cell carcinoma
  Kaposi's sarcoma
  Initiating factors (if any)

Diagnosis:
  History: duration, scabbing bleeding, pain, itching
  Site and size
  Appearance: surface, edges, base
  Histology
  Regional lymphadenopathy

Treatment:
  Surgical: wide local excision (except Kaposi's sarcoma)
  Block dissection of involved regional nodes
  Adjuvant: radio-, chemo- and immunotherapies

Prognosis:
  Dependent on type, histological grading and spread (nodal/visceral)

Follow up:
  Long term for all except rodent ulcer
  Treatment of recurrences

Question 2

Write an essay on the management of a 36-year-old man who sustained a spinal injury at C7–T1 level in a riding accident.

Plan

Immediate measures:

    Primary survey:

        airway maintenance

        BP, pulse and respiratory monitoring

        neurological assessment

        resuscitation

    Secondary survey: detailed physical examination

Assessment of injuries:

    Neurological deficits

    Associated injuries

Treatment:

    Surgical: stabilise spinal fracture/dislocation

    Supportive: maintenance of bodily function:

        nutrition

        bladder

        bowel

Monitor recovery of neurological function

Avoid morbidity: bed sores, bone demineralisation, muscle atrophy

Physiotherapy: maximise functional recovery by exercise regimens and physical aids

Community care: adjustments to home/work environment

Long-term complications of paraplegia

Question 3

A 30-year-old woman presents with an asymptomatic lump in her left breast. Discuss your clinical assessment and management.

Plan

Working diagnosis on history and clinical features

Investigations:

  Mammography/ultrasonography

  Fine-needle aspiration biopsy (FNAB)

  Biopsy (excisional/incisional)

  Further investigations: chest radiograph, bone and liver scans, if indicated

Definitive diagnosis from above

Counselling of patient

Treatment:

Surgical:

  benign: local excision

  malignant: mastectomy (segmental or total)

  axillary dissection

Adjuvant therapy:

  based on histological type and spread:

  regional deep X-ray therapy

  tamoxifen

  chemotherapy

  endocrine ablation (oophorectomy, adrenalectomy, hypophysectomy)

Follow-up:

  Long-term (annual after 5 years' recurrence free)

  Diagnosis, restaging and treatment of recurrent disease

Question 4

Write an essay on the causes, presentation and treatment of obstructive jaundice.

Plan

Causes:

    Congenital: biliary atresia

    Inflammatory: sclerosing cholangitis

    Infective: ascending cholangitis; parasitic (round) worms

    Metabolic: duct stones or sludge

    Iatrogenic: bile duct injury

    Neoplastic: cholangiocarcinoma; periampulatory carcinoma, metastatic spread to lymph nodes in the porta hepatis

Presentation:

    Symptoms: weakness, wasting, loss of appetite, fever, itchiness, pale stools

    Signs: jaundice, hepatomegaly, ascites, palpable gallbladder

Treatment:

    Relief of obstruction: by percutaneous transhepatic drainage and cholangiogram and/or ERCP to identify lesion

    Antibiotic therapy on bile culture

    Surgical measures:

        duct exploration, resection, biliary bypass

        endoscopic stenting with/without chemotherapy for inoperable lesions

Question 5

Write an essay on the causation and the diagnosis of blood in the urine in a 70-year-old man.

Plan

Causes:

  Kidneys: acute nephritis, stone, tumour

  Ureter: stone, tumour

  Bladder: acute cystitis, polyps, tumour, stone (schistosomiasis)

  Prostate: tumour, prostatic surgery

  Urethra: stone

  Unknown aetiology

History:

  Duration of haematuria

  Blood mixed in urine or appears at start/end of micturition

  Stranguary

  Abdominal symptoms

Clinical findings:

  General: pallor, BP, pulse

  Renal/bladder mass

  Prostatic enlargement irregularity

  Urethral lesion

Investigations:

  FBC, U&Es

  MSU (midstream urine specimen) to confirm haematuria and to test for sugar

  Ultrasonography of kidneys/bladder

  IVU

  If the above are negative/normal: repeat urinary microscopy

  If haematuria persists: ureteric catheterisation for selective urine samples

  Renal imaging

  Once lesion is identified: histological confirmation by endoscopic biopsy or FNAB under imaging

Question 6

Write an essay on the causation, presentation and treatment of small bowel obstruction.

Plan

Causes:

    Intraluminal: bolus obstruction

    In bowel wall: lymphoid hyperplasia and tumours leading to intussusception, vascular occlusion (mesenteric infarction)

    Extraneous: internal herniations; external hernias

    Iatrogenic: surgical adhesions or incisional hernias

Presentation:

    Symptoms and signs of complete/incomplete obstruction: vomiting, dehydration, constipation, colic, abdominal signs

    Previous episodes/operations/outcomes

    Characteristics of palpable mass or visible peristalsis

    Signs of bowel ischaemia

Abdominal radiograph: erect and supine:

    Air–fluid levels, level of obstruction from the configuration of proximal distended loops

Treatment:

    Nasogastric suction

    Rehydrate, electrolyte replacement

    Urgent surgical relief of obstruction, except in adhesion obstruction when non-surgical measures are continued

    Repair of causative hernia at same time

Question

Write an essay on the presentation and management of chronic arterial disease of the lower limb.

Answer 1: A comfortable pass

Introduction
Chronic arterial disease afflicting the aorta, the iliacs and the vessels in the lower limb may produce stenosis, occlusion or aneurysmal dilatation. Atherosclerosis is the common vascular lesion and may also involve coronary, cerebral and renal arteries. Association risk factors are diabetes mellitus, hypertension, smoking, raised blood lipid levels and a family history of vascular disease.

Symptoms and signs
Stenosis of the main arteries reduces the blood flow to the lower limb, producing intermittent claudication as a result of temporary muscle ischaemia: the claudication distance is the distance that the patient is able to walk before stopping. Rest pain in the limb indicates severe restriction to blood flow, which is inadequate for resting tissue metabolism. The pain is characteristically in the foot, worse at night and relieved by dangling the limb out of bed or sleeping in a chair. Pain referred to the limb from degenerative disease of the lumbosacral spine, the hip or the knee, or caused by peripheral neuropathy, must be distinguished from ischaemic pain.

Coldness, numbness and paraesthesiae are present with skin pallor on elevation of and duskiness on lowering the limb. Buerger's angle is the angle of elevation at which blanching first occurs and is accompanied by venous emptying or, in severe ischaemia, venous guttering. The time taken for the veins to refill on hanging the limb down indicates the extent of vascular compromise. In severe ischaemia the skin may be mottled and without sensation. Occasionally, symptoms and signs of acute-on-chronic ischaemia develop.

Ulceration occurs with severe arterial insufficiency and presents as painful, indolent, nonhealing ulcers in the toes or pressure areas in the foot and occasionally over the ankle or the shin. Arterial pulses are reduced or absent distal to the diseased artery, and occasionally a thrill or a bruit may be detected over the latter, caused by turbulent flow.

The presence of a pulsatile and expansile swelling in the abdomen indicates an aortic aneurysm, whereas a femoral or a popliteal aneurysm may be felt in the groin or behind the knee. They may be asymptomatic but can present with acute rupture or thrombosis.

Investigations
The severity of the symptoms determines the need for vascular investigations, and non-invasive ultrasound tests are performed routinely on presentation. The ankle brachial pressure index (ABPI) is the ratio of systolic pressure in the ankle to that in the arm. The normal is 1.0. In people with claudication the resting index is usually < 1.0 and falls below the resting value after exercise. A resting index of = 0.5 indicates critical ischaemia. The results of noninvasive tests indicate the need for further assessment with a view to treatment. Angiography by conventional or digital techniques demonstrates the anatomical site or sites and the severity of the disease process, and enables treatment to be planned.

Treatment

Most claudicants require only reassurance and advice about weight reduction, low-fat diet and stopping smoking, as appropriate. Intercurrent diseases, such as diabetes and hypertension, must be actively treated. Daily exercise regimens to improve the blood supply by developing collateral circulations must be actively encouraged. Foot care is essential to avoid injury to skin that may already be compromised. A daily aspirin tablet (75 mg) improves tissue perfusion by lowering the blood viscosity.

In the presence of incapacitating claudication or rest pain, transluminal angioplasty is used as the first line of treatment. It dilates the stenosed lumen with an inflatable balloon introduced on an arterial catheter under fluoroscopic screening. Intraluminal stents may occasionally be inserted to keep the lumen open after dilatation.

Surgery for occlusive disease is indicated when angioplasty is not feasible. Aortic or aortoiliac disease may be bypassed with a Dacron tube or bifurcation graft; in the case of aortic or iliac aneurysm the sac is opened and the graft sutured in. When intra-abdominal surgery is contraindicated, grafts are placed from the ipsilateral axillary or the contralateral common femoral arteries.

Arterial narrowing below the inguinal ligament is bypassed using the long saphenous vein. In its absence a PTFE graft is used, and to prolong its patency a collar of vein is interposed between the distal end of the graft and the recipient artery. Aneurysms in the limb are similarly bypassed and excluded from the circulation to prevent emboli from the clot present within them. Skin perfusion may be improved by lumbar sympathectomy when revascularisation is not feasible.

Clinical and sonographic surveillance is important in monitoring graft patency and impending graft occlusion. With progressive deterioration in symptoms, amputation of the limb should be considered with a planned rehabilitation programme aimed at restoring mobility. This includes physiotherapy and involvement of occupational therapists to ensure that home conditions are appropriate for discharge from hospital.

Examiner's comments on Answer 1
- The essay is eminently readable, knowledgeable and concise, with appropriate subdivisions.
- The introduction defines the problem and gives emphasis to atherosclerosis with its risk factors.
- Diagnosis is based on the history, examination and investigations, and the candidate has commented on the relevant points in each group.
- The question is very broad and, therefore, treatment can be covered only in outline. Clear guidelines on each treatment modality are stated.
- Emphasis is given to the conservative management of most patients, and medical management available is outlined.
- The importance of angioplasty is given as the first line of management, and the main forms of surgical intervention are summarised.
- The importance of follow up is stated.
- The possible need for amputation is noted, together with the necessary team work for subsequent rehabilitation.

Answer 2: An Answer Showing Inadequate Knowledge

The aetiology of chronic arterial disease of the lower limbs is poor general health resulting from various organic disease states and poor lifestyle. Presentation may be divided into symptoms and signs. The classic symptom of chronic arterial disease of the lower limb is pain. This may be constant or intermittent, and described as affecting mainly the feet or the entire limb, but the most usual presentation is intermittent claudication, this being a sharp pain affecting one or both calves that is induced by exercise and relieved by rest. It is often more troublesome in cold weather. The amount of exercise necessary to bring on the pain is extremely variable but the most troublesome confounding factor in eliciting a history of claudication is the coexistence of osteoarthritis, which may make exercise painful and even mask the presence of arterial disease by precluding walking on its own account. Pain may also arise as a result of ulceration and the patient may complain of cold legs. In late-stage disease a blackened toe may be the presentation.

Although pain is a feature of ischaemia, tissue that has died is anaesthetic, and manipulation of areas of gangrene may cause severe pain at the granulating demarcation between living and dead tissue. Patients with chronic disease may occasionally present acutely, with complete cessation of blood flow secondary to thrombus formation, leading to paralysis of the limb which becomes pale, paraesthetic and cold with undetectable pulses or life-threatening gas gangrene, where the patient is systemically ill and the offending limb is pale or green, and malodorous and may exhibit the characteristic 'crackling' sensation of gas in the tissues on examination.

Signs of chronic arterial disease of the lower limb include loss of hair, cool skin, ulcers that are characteristically small and well demarcated, pulses that are difficult or impossible to palpate, blackened extremities and stumps that are sites of previous amputations. The femoral pulses should always be auscultated because bruits will often be heard. The management of chronic arterial disease may be divided into investigations, medical and surgical treatment, nursing and physiotherapy. Various radiological investigations may be performed. Such investigations may include angiography, whereas MRI (magnetic resonance imaging) may make a big impact on angiography in the future by allowing digital subtraction images to be constructed non-invasively. Medical treatment will almost always include an anti-clotting agent, such as aspirin, typically 75 mg once daily. Treatment of coexisting medical illness, particularly coronary artery disease, should not be overlooked. A number of drugs are available to promote arterial dilatation in the peripheries.

Surgical intervention may include endarterectomy if the lesion is relatively localised and in an accessible position. Bypass grafts using PTFE tubing are most useful for restoring blood supply. They may be done at various levels and the femoropopliteal graft is the classic operation. Surgical treatment often involves amputation if conservative treatment of areas of gangrenous tissue fails. Amputation requires a balance between leaving as much viable tissue as possible and ensuring that the tissue left remains viable;

patients are often medically so ill that reoperation is even more undesirable than usual. Nursing care includes care of the whole patient, dressing of ulcers, and scrupulous attention to hygiene on areas of tissue that may have died or are of dubious viability. Physiotherapy may improve the function of existing limbs and aid familiarisation with artificial limbs, crutches, etc.

Examiner's comments on Answer 2
Reads well, with many common-sense statements, but:
- Introduction limited to a vague statement, with no mention of risk factors
- No subheadings
- Inadequate paragraphs
- Too much emphasis given to osteoarthritis and gas gangrene, which have little relevance to the question set
- Pain affects the 'entire limb'
- Nutrition and postural changes in the foot are missing
- No mention of non-invasive tests, namely pressure measurements, imaging or waveform analysis
- No mention of indications for angiography
- No mention of drugs, such as antiplatelet agents and their limitations, and percutaneous transluminal angioplasty (PTA) – the current first choice of therapeutic measure
- No mention of aorto-iliac disease
- No mention of extra-anatomical bypass or the limitations of synthetic grafts across the knee
- The importance of amputations was mentioned, but no occupational therapy or rehabilitation of the amputee.

PART FOUR

Essay Questions

Essay Questions

I. Surgical Physiology

1. Discuss the principles of postoperative fluid and electrolyte balance.

2. Describe the preparation of a patient for an abdominal operation and the immediate postoperative management.

3. What is meant by circulatory collapse and shock? List the causes and describe how you would treat one of them.

4. Discuss the investigation and management of a patient who is alleged to have a 'bleeding tendency' before and after major surgery.

II. Trauma and Burns

1. A 14-year-old boy is admitted to the Emergency Department with right-sided abdominal pain, after falling 5 metres (15 feet) from a tree. Discuss your assessment and treatment.

2. Describe the priorities of diagnosis and management in a severely injured person.

3. A 10-year-old girl lacerated her wrist on a plate glass window. Describe the structures that may be damaged, indicating how such damage may be diagnosed and treated.

4. Write an essay on the management of skin burns.

5. Discuss the management of a 23-year-old man who was crushed when the seating terrace collapsed at a football stadium.

III. Orthopaedics

1. Discuss the management of a 67-year-old woman with osteoarthritis of the hip.

2. A young man was seen in the orthopaedic clinic with a painful swollen knee after a rotational football injury 3 days previously. Discuss the diagnosis and outline your management.

3. Describe the management and potential complications in a 65-year-old woman with a compound fracture of the tibia and fibula.

4. Write an essay on the diagnosis and treatment of fractures of the femur in an adult.

5. An 80-year-old woman complains of pain in her thoracic spine. Discuss the differential diagnoses and the management of the most common cause of such a symptom.

IV. Neurosurgery

1. Write an essay on the assessment and treatment of an adult patient admitted unconscious after a road traffic accident.

2. Describe the various types of peripheral nerve injuries and how you would evaluate and treat them.

3. Describe the common forms of spina bifida and discuss its complications and treatment.
   Or
   Write an essay on hydrocephalus and its management.

V. Skin, Eyes and ENT

1. Discuss the diagnosis and management of a 36-year-old woman with a malignant melanoma of the skin over her calf.

2. A young man presents to the Emergency Department with discomfort and hazy vision in one eye a few hours after working with a hammer and chisel. What are the possible findings? Discuss the investigations and treatment that may be indicated.

3. Describe the causes of a painful red eye and the management of this condition.

4. Discuss the clinical presentation, the complications and treatment of chronic suppurative otitis media.

5. Describe the causes and discuss the management of a patient with a severe nosebleed.

VI. Endocrinology, Breast and Chest

1. Write an essay on the disorders that may arise from abnormalities of the adrenal glands and their surgical treatment.

2. Describe the diagnosis and management of a 40-year-old woman who presents with a solitary nodule in the left lobe of the thyroid.

3. Discuss the diagnosis and management of a 35-year-old woman presenting with a painless lump in the breast.

4. List the causes and discuss the diagnosis and management of a patient with a pneumothorax.

5. Write an essay on the presentation, aetiology, investigation and treatment of a carcinoma of the bronchus.

6. Write an essay on the investigation and interventional and surgical measures used in treating ischaemic heart disease.

VII. Upper Alimentary Tract

1. A 64-year-old man presents with a 3-month history of increasing difficulty in swallowing solid food. Discuss the diagnosis and management of this patient.

2. Write an essay on the diagnosis and treatment of haematemesis in a 56-year-old woman.

3. Discuss the surgical causes of vomiting in a 14-day-old neonate. Describe how you would diagnose and treat one such condition.

4. Discuss the diagnosis and management of a patient with a perforated peptic ulcer.

5. Write an essay on the indications for splenectomy and the complications of this procedure.

VIII. Liver, Gallbladder and Pancreas

1. Write an essay on the diagnosis and treatment of a patient suffering from acute cholecystitis.

2. Discuss the presentation, the diagnosis and management of a 68-year-old man with obstructive jaundice.

3. Write an essay on portal hypertension and its management.

4. Discuss the causes of liver abscess and its treatment.

5. Write an essay on the aetiology, diagnosis and management of acute pancreatitis.

IX. Small and Large Bowel

1. Discuss the diagnosis and management of a 32-year-old man who presents with a painful, tender mass in the right iliac fossa.

2. Discuss the aetiology and complications of diverticulitis of the colon. Describe the clinical features of the disease and the principles of treatment.

3. Write an essay on the differential diagnosis and management of a 65-year-old woman complaining of left lower abdominal pain and constipation of 10 weeks' duration.

4. An 18-month-old boy said to be suffering from abdominal colic passed blood-stained mucus per rectum. Discuss the diagnosis and management.

X. Urology

1. Describe the clinical presentation and management of a patient with a hypernephroma (Grawitz's tumour).

2. Describe the management of an adult presenting with haematuria.

3. Describe the types of undescended testis, its treatment and complications.

4. A 35-year-old man presented to the surgical clinic with a hard, painless swelling of the scrotum. Describe the management of this patient.

5. Write an essay on urethral stricture in an adult male.

XI. Vascular Surgery

1. Describe the causes, presentation and management of an embolus of the femoral artery in a 50-year-old woman seen within 6 hours of the onset of symptoms.

2. A 61-year-old man presents to the surgical clinic with a 9-month history of pain in his right calf that occurs after walking 100 metres on the flat, and is relieved by rest. Discuss the diagnosis and management of this patient and the factors that would influence the latter.

3. Discuss the causes and describe the management of gangrene of the toes.

4. Discuss the management of a 70-year-old man presenting with an asymptomatic, pulsatile and expansile mass in the abdomen.

5. Discuss the aetiology and management of lower leg ulceration.

APPENDIX A

The Final Examination in Surgery

Assessment of clinical competence

Medical training encompasses a wide range of complex and varied activities and has evolved to match the diverse abilities required of the practising clinician. Maintaining these skills is essential for the establishment of professional standards of excellence and satisfying public expectation.

Assessment of clinical competence over such a broad field is fraught with difficulty: it has to examine the results of a number of years of study, covering a large syllabus in a uniform, efficient, competent and reliable fashion. It should ensure that candidates who have achieved the required level of proficiency pass, and those who have not should fail. The examination should be seen, by students and examiners, as being fair.

The perfect examination has not only to assess knowledge and understanding accurately but also to evaluate the powers of analysis in problem-solving and decision-making. In the clinical field the candidate's attitude to patients and clinical work, as well as their personal and professional development and conduct, must also be evaluated.

Why examine?

Over the last few decades a number of groups have questioned the need for formal assessment and have proposed continuous, faculty-based evaluation in medical education. Nevertheless, the vast majority of medical schools and universities rely on staged examinations to ensure the acquisition of a minimal knowledge base. Satisfactory performance may be accompanied by graduation, certification and the right to practise. The level of achievement may influence progress and promotion.

Examinations are also valuable for students and teachers to establish personal and departmental standards, and one of the problems of statutory examinations is usually their lack of feedback of the details of a candidate's performance. Internal faculty examinations can be an aid to learning and a means of self-evaluation: this will become of increasing importance with the extension of continued medical education, to help students identify a weakness of both personal knowledge and teaching material. Even the most ardent supporters of continuous assessment cannot deny the stimulus and motivation of an examination, and it does separate good from bad candidates.

What system?

To justify their existence, examinations have to be seen as fair and linked with both the training and its stated objectives. Traditional medical examinations have been based on the essay, the oral and the clinical. History and examination are central to a doctor–patient relationship, and the clinical has held its ground in undergraduate and postgraduate assessment (although the division between medicine and surgery, and other disciplines has often become blurred, the emphasis being on the history and examination rather than the underlying disorder). Short cases in some schools have been replaced or supplemented by Objective Structured Clinical Examinations (OSCEs) to accompany the written part, and orals have been restricted to distinction and borderline candidates.

The essay has come under the greatest scrutiny. Students and examiners have questioned the effectiveness of an essay paper, because the limited number of topics and the possible choices have encouraged students to spot questions and concentrate on only part of the syllabus. The marking of essays is time-consuming and unreliable. There may be variation in the individual examiner's reassessment of papers, as well as between examiners. The

APPENDIX A

variation makes comparison at a national level difficult, and this is further accentuated by what has been described as the deep psychological reluctance of examiners to allocate more than 70% of the total marks allowed for any given essay question.

Attempts to modify the essay included modified essay questions (MEQs), introducing a larger number of questions with a patient vignette, and a variety of subsections based on various aspects of diagnosis and treatment. Multiple short answers on a range of topics have also gained favour in some schools. Structured answer questions (SAQs) are a further development of the written assessment, testing problem-solving and decision-making in a structured and objective fashion. They are proving a reliable means of assessing knowledge and understanding in clinical practice.

MCQs also have a wide application in medical assessment, having the potential to cover a wide body of knowledge and, in their extended matching pairs format, introducing reasoned responses rather than item recall. A computerised marking system has eased the examiners' burden in this section. A current trend in the written part of the clinical examination is to include both MCQs and SAQs, the former to determine the candidate's knowledge and the latter to assess the application of this knowledge by reasoning, interpretation, problem-solving and decision-making.

SAQs

SAQs test the candidate's high-level skills rather than factual recall. They consist of a clinical vignette followed by two to four questions, which may have subsections, with an indication of the marks allocated for each correct answer. The choice of scenario is based on common clinical problems pertinent and relevant to the field of study, and covering important concepts and principles relating to the course material. There is no room for trivia, irrelevant or esoteric topics, or interesting rarities.

Clinical information is presented in an ordered fashion, usually describing the history and examination, with or without investigations, of a specific condition. Questions should be clear, unambiguous and requiring the examinee to analyse and make decisions based on the given information. This may involve diagnosis or treatment and may also cover aspects of psychological, social and family history, and ethical issues.

Examiners are given a model answer and a marking schedule that has to be closely adhered to. Marking is time-consuming: allotting a single examiner to each question streamlines the process and allows uniformity of marking for a group of candidates. Any allowances made for near misses will also be generalised. It is common to double mark a number of scripts to check examiners' interobserver reliability across the whole examination.

Examiners preparing SAQs should form a panel, draw up a list of topics and allocate these topics among the group. The first draft of each question is read out at a group meeting, and comments made on the content, style, importance and relevance, and its educational standard.

The second draft of the questions is tried on a group of students under examination conditions, noting the time taken to complete four to eight questions. The answers are analysed and questions again modified if there are obvious misunderstandings, or unexpected ease or difficulty.

Misinterpretation of the stem may lead to an erroneous diagnosis. As the rest of the question is usually based on the stem, a candidate may go off at a tangent in all subsequent answers. The examiners must then make an informed decision in allocating marks for such mishaps, provided that the conclusions reached are logical and not far removed from the expected answers. However, in inadequately vetted questions more than one diagnosis may be arrived at from the stem. In such circumstances the onus is firmly on the examiner to accommodate such unanticipated correct responses and mark them fairly.

The completed questions are retained in a question bank. They should be added to each year, attention being given to the choice, number and range of topics. These should match the weighting given to each part of the syllabus. It may take 3–5 years to build up an adequate bank; after this time any break in security is of less importance.

APPENDIX A

The stem of a question can often be modified by changing the disease and superficial data, such as the sex, age and timing of the symptoms. This process eases the generation of further questions and allows some degree of comparison of standards when they are being analysed. Questions should be under continuous reappraisal after each use, to assess their performance and discriminatory value. Marks can be influenced by poor quality questions, poor knowledge of answers and errors within the marking system. Each examination requires 10–12 questions to allow a broad assessment and to produce discriminatory differences between good and bad candidates. Each question used should be independent of the others.

Essays

MCQs are used routinely in most qualifying and postgraduate examinations. Nevertheless, medicine is not as black and white as MCQs would suggest, and many brighter students are averse to this form of assessment. Similarly, although SAQs allow much wider coverage of the syllabus and more objectivity in the marking systems, they also restrict the examiner to black-and-white rigid marking schemes. The limitations of these features are well known to every clinician who has gone over recent examinations with groups of students.

The essay does test a candidate's ability to collect and quantify material, and assesses powers of original thought and creativity. It determines the candidate's ability to write clear and legible English, and some schools have felt that these qualities should be retained in their assessment. In spite of the expensive manpower required in marking essay questions, an essay does assess a candidate's depth of knowledge in a specified area and, in preparing for an essay paper, candidates have to acquire detailed knowledge of much of the syllabus.

Revision for the essay paper is linked with revision of the whole course. If a candidate's knowledge base is poor, he or she will rightly fail, but, even if it is sound, good examination technique is essential for success. The ease of revision is based on previous knowledge and a good filing system which, if disease based, provides a checklist for each condition, so that current knowledge can be written and then checked against books and stored material to identify deficiencies.

The candidate is expected to have read around topics and patient problems encountered during the clinical course, gaining information from lectures, reviews and current papers, as well as textbooks. This information should be filed in an easily retrievable form, such as notes in the margins of textbooks, a card system, plenty of lists and clearly written pieces of paper. This in turn is transcribed (or transferred directly) onto one's personal electronic files for future use. People vary in the amount of information that they can remember at any one time. Any deficiency, however, can be easily reversed during revision, provided that previous information was well organised and fully understood at the time that it was collected.

Examiners at an undergraduate level are keen to pass candidates, to ensure that they can continue with their careers. However, medical examiners have an obligation to ensure that ignorant and potentially dangerous individuals are not let loose on a patient population. At a postgraduate level examiners have to ensure that a candidate has a comprehensive and indepth knowledge of their subject: gaps are likely to be penalised.

Regardless of the level of the examination, essays on clinical subjects have a similar format. This is based on a disease or a clinical problem and includes questions on the aetiology, pathology, diagnosis, differential diagnoses, complications, assessment, management and treatment. Each question must be read carefully and every word noted, because they will have been constructed very carefully.

Although the words 'discuss' and a few synonyms imply a certain vagueness, the response must be precise and directed. Having read the question, the answer plan is based on the clinical data required. These will usually correspond to the checklist used to revise each disease.

Diagnosis and differential diagnoses are based on only three sources of information: namely, the **history**, **examination** and

APPENDIX A

investigation. If the diagnosis is given, it may require confirmation from the same three sources. Assessment means diagnosis (history, examination, investigation), but adds the dimension of severity of the problems encountered. Management is assessment plus treatment. Although the term may be used loosely, implying just treatment in some questions, it is worth writing a few sentences on confirmation of the diagnosis and the severity of the problem being treated. Treatment should not be restricted to surgery, because many other problems may need to be sorted out first.

Other disciplines that may be involved must be considered, such as nursing, physiotherapy, occupational therapy, and drugs, chemotherapeutic agents and radiotherapy. Radiological intervention forms a major part of treatment in many diseases.

The plan outlining the areas to be covered can be in the answer book or on scrap paper. The plan should take 3–6 minutes for most essays and allows concentrated thought around the topic. On completion, a line is drawn through it to imply to the examiner that there is more to come, and the first few sentences of the introduction are constructed. This should imply an understanding of the topic, giving the examiner confidence that the essay is on the right track, and, hopefully, is of good standard.

There is much debate about whether headings should be underlined and key words highlighted. This debate is more of a problem to the candidate than to the examiner, who is more concerned about whether a script is legible and demonstrates knowledge and understanding of the question. Illegibility is an inherent problem with some individuals. Examiners go to considerable effort to give candidates the benefit of the doubt but illegibility can never camouflage ignorance, and candidates would be well advised to write at a rate at which the end product is guaranteed to be readable to the examiner.

Literacy and mastery of prose are more debatable. As much as examiners would wish medical graduates to be able to write skilfully and coherently, marks are predominantly awarded for factual knowledge and understanding of an essay topic. Success is, therefore, based on an appropriate plan and the development of each heading within it.

Medical schools and surgical colleges rarely set regular essays during their courses, even when they use this means of final assessment. It is, therefore, appropriate for students who know that they will be examined in this way to undertake preliminary practice. A series of essay questions has, therefore, been added after the SAQ sections. There is a section on planned structural outlines as a preliminary to writing essays and examples of good and poor answers with examiner's comments. These guidelines may be used to plan and write essays. The relevant practical information will usually be found in the sectional answers and teaching aids, and essays may be swapped with a working partner or discussion group, who would act as examiners. Subsequently, the plan, development, depth of knowledge, literary style and legibility are discussed. As the finals draw near, the pass standard becomes apparent and essays can be accurately assessed by peer review.

Whichever examination system is chosen, it must be reliable, valid and discriminatory, and it should not be influenced by the subjective judgement of an examiner. The examination should be about the contents of a paper and not expertise or prior coaching in the chosen system. Nevertheless, it is essential to have prior exposure to the local examination system and be well versed in its technique. This text is intended to provide that exposure and to educate candidates in the techniques of SAQ and essay writing in the hope of easing their passage to qualification.

Self-assessment SAQ Papers

Notes for Readers – SAQ Exam Papers

There are 12 questions in each paper, to be answered in 2 hours.
- You are advised to spend no more than 10 minutes on each question.
- The questions are designed to promote succinct answers.
- The marks awarded for each section are indicated.

Paper 1: 1.4, 2.1, 3.5, 3.6, 4.4, 5.5, 6.1, 7.2, 8.2, 9.4, 10.4, 11.1
Paper 2: 1.5, 2.2, 2.14, 3.7, 4.5, 5.6, 6.7, 7.3, 8.3, 9.5, 10.5, 11.2
Paper 3: 1.1, 2.11, 3.2, 3.8, 5.2, 5.7, 6.14, 7.4, 8.4, 9.10, 10.6, 11.3
Paper 4: 1.6, 2.4, 3.9, 4.7, 5.8, 6.8, 7.5, 8.5, 9.7, 10.7, 10.14, 11.5
Paper 5: 1.7, 2.16, 3.15, 4.8, 5.9, 6.3, 6.12, 7.11, 8.6, 9.8, 10.9, 11.6
Paper 6: 1.8, 2.6, 3.11, 4.9, 5.10, 6.6, 6.9, 7.8, 8.7, 9.9, 10.10, 11.7
Paper 7: 1.9, 2.7, 2.13, 3.4, 3.16, 5.11, 6.10, 7.5, 7.6, 8.8, 10.11, 11.8
Paper 8: 1.2, 2.5, 3.10, 4.6, 5.12, 6.2, 7.4, 7.7, 8.9, 9.2, 10.12, 11.9
Paper 9: 1.10, 2.8, 2.10, 3.12, 4.2, 5.4, 6.4, 7.3, 9.6, 9.12, 10.8, 10.13
Paper 10: 2.3, 2.15, 3.1, 4.10, 5.1, 6.11, 7.1, 8.1, 9.1, 10.1, 10.2, 11.11
Paper 11: 1.3, 2.9, 2.12, 3.3, 5.3, 6.5, 6.13, 7.6, 9.3, 10.3, 11.4, 10.13
Paper 12: 1.11, 2.18, 3.18, 4.11, 5.12, 5.15, 6.4, 7.8, 8.12, 8.13, 12.1, 12.12

APPENDIX C

Self-assessment Essay Question Papers

Notes for Readers – Essay Exam Questions

There are four questions in each paper, to be answered in 2 hours.
- You are advised to spend no more than 30 minutes on each question and to spend the first 5 minutes formulating an outline for your answer.

Paper 1: 2.1, 4.1, 6.1, 8.1
Paper 2: 1.2, 2.2, 9.2, 11.2
Paper 3: 1.3, 2.3, 6.3, 10.3
Paper 4: 2.4, 5.4, 9.4, 11.4
Paper 5: 2.5, 5.5, 6.2, 8.2
Paper 6: 1.4, 3.1, 7.1, 10.5
Paper 7: 3.2, 5.3, 7.2, 11.1
Paper 8: 3.3, 4.2, 7.3, 8.3
Paper 9: 3.4, 6.4, 7.4, 10.4
Paper 10: 4.3, 9.3, 10.2, 11.3
Paper 11: 3.5, 5.1, 6.5, 7.7
Paper 12: 1.1, 5.2, 9.1, 10.1

Index of Cases

(The number in bold indicates the section and the number in italics indicates the case number.)